Dedication

I dedicate this book to my loving, belated father whose kind words of encouragement and support have helped me through my most challenging times. He will be always remembered and his memories cherished.

Surgical Specialities
MCQ Series

PLASTIC SURGERY

QUIZ

A COLLECTION OF 500 MCQ AND EMQ QUESTIONS

D. Oudit
MB.,BS, FRCSEd(Plast)
Consultant Plastic and Reconstructive Surgeon
The Christie Hospital NHS Foundation Trust
Manchester, UK
Honorary Senior Lecturer
University of Manchester

Surgical Specialities
MCQ Series

PLASTIC SURGERY

QUIZ

A COLLECTION OF 500 MCQ AND EMQ QUESTIONS

Copyright © 2015 by Surgicalillustration.com

All rights reserved. No part of this book may be reproduced or transmitted in any form or by any means without written permission from the author.

ISBN 978-0-9574996-3-8

TABLE OF CONTENTS

Preface..7

Quiz 1..9

Quiz 2...34

Quiz 3...60

Quiz 4...86

Quiz 5..111

Quiz 6..137

Quiz 7..163

Quiz 8..190

Quiz 9..216

Quiz 10...242

Acknowledgements

I would like to sincerely thank my wife for her continuous and unwavering support during the course of completing this project.

I would also to thank Matthew Briggs, Senior Medical Artist for preparing the illustrations for this book.

Preface

The final FRCS(Plast) and the American National Board Exams can be challenging at the best of times. One of the best exam preparation techniques is to practice using questions that are pitched at the level of the exams and covering the whole breadth of the speciality.

This work, Plastic Surgery Quiz, is a collection of 500 multiple choice (MCQs) and extended matching (EMQs) questions. It is the first in a series of revision books for the major surgical specialities.

The questions are arranged into 10 quizzes, each covering the wide breadth of the speciality. Each quiz comprises of 40 MCQs and 10 EMQs. The answers are presented at the end of each quiz with brief explanations and extra study material.

This book is suitable for plastic surgery trainees and plastic surgery residents revising or preparing for their final exits exams or the National Board Exams. It would also be suitable as a revision aid covering a wide range of topics within Plastic Surgery.

We hope that you would find it useful as a revision tool.

Best wishes,

DO

Manchester, UK
2015

QUIZ 1
MULTIPLE CHOICE QUESTIONS

For questions 1.1 to 1.40 please the ONE most appropriate answer.

Q 1.1

A 25 year-old male patient has a 20 x 20cm puckered scar on the right side of his back following a flame burn 2 years ago. The full-thickness burn wound was managed conservatively by regular dressings. Which ONE of the following functions is not altered by the scar compared to the surrounding normal skin?

[A] Thermoregulation

[B] Sensation

[C] Protection against microbiological invasion

[D] Protection against ultraviolet light

Q 1.2

Which of the following statements is FALSE with regards to the structure of the epidermis?

[A] The skin of the back is thick because it has a relatively thick stratum lucidum

[B] Actively proliferating cells are only present on the basal layer of the epidermis

[C] Melanocytes are present in the basal layer

[D] Squamous cell carcinomas arise from the stratum spinosum of the epidermis

Q 1.3

Which one of the following types of cells is NOT present in the epidermis in normal healthy skin?

[A] Langerhan's cells

[B] Fibroblasts

[C] Merkel cells

[D] Melanocytes

Q 1.4
During the inflammatory phase of wound healing, vasodilation is mediated by all of the following compounds EXCEPT?

[A] Histamine

[B] Thromboxane

[C] Serotonin

[D] Nitrous oxide

Q 1.5
Which of the following events does NOT occur in the remodelling phase of wound healing?

[A] Proliferation of capillaries

[B] Collagen fibre rearrangement

[C] No net increase or decrease in the amount of collagen in the wound

[D] Restoration of the relative proportions of Type 1 and Type 3 collagen

Q 1.6
Prolongation of which of the following phases of wound may result in a hypertrophic scar?

[A] Haemostasis

[B] Inflammation

[C] Proliferation

[D] Remodelling

Q 1.7
Which of the following is NOT a characteristic of laser light?

[A] It is monochromatic

[B] It is produced by a chromophore

[C] It is collimated

[D] It is coherent

Q 1.8
Tissue expanded skin has which one of the following properties?

[A] Utilises the elastic properties of the skin and therefore there are no new cells in the expanded tissue

[B] All of the expanded skin is composed of new cells

[C] Has an improved blood supply compared to surrounding normal skin

[D] Is asensate

Q 1.9
Which of the following is the MOST common craniofacial cleft?

[A] Cleft no. 3

[B] Cleft no. 6

[C] Cleft No. 7

[D] Cleft no. 8

Q 1.10
Which of the following cranial suture is the first to fuse?

[A] Lambdoid suture

[B] Sagittal suture

[C] Coronal suture

[D] Metopic suture

Q 1.11
Which of the following is a feature of allografts?

[A] Tissue derived from a different species

[B] Non-living tissue derived from a member of the same species

[C] Non-living tissue derived from a member of a different species

[D] Preserved non-living tissue derived from the same individual

Q 1.12
What is the mechanism resulting in the cleft primary palate?

[A] Failure of fusion of the lateral nasal process with the maxillary process

[B] Failure of fusion of the medial nasal process with the mandibular process

[C] Failure of fusion of the medial nasal process with the maxillary process

[D] Failure of fusion of the palatal shelves

Q 1.13
Which geographical location has the highest incidence of cleft lip and palate?

[A] Europe

[B] Scandinavia

[C] Africa

[D] Asia

Q 1.14
Which of the following statements regarding giant congenital hairy naevii is TRUE?

[A] Histologically, they are confined to the epidermis

[B] They remain the same size from birth and characteristically do not grow in proportion to the body size

[C] They are benign lesions and do not carry any risk of malignant transformation

[D] They are not confined to the dermis and may invade into underlying muscle and bone

Q 1.15
Which of the following is NOT a cardinal feature of sarcomas?

[A] Pain associated with the lesion

[B] Size of lesion > 5cm

[C] Associated with a leukocytosis

[D] Lesion deep to fascia

Q 1.16
Which one of the following is NOT a well-recognised feature of Gorlins syndrome?

[A] Large head circumference

[B] Cardiac fibromas

[C] Mental retardation

[D] Palmar pits

Q 1.17
With regards to Photodynamic therapy is TRUE?

[A] It is a useful modality of treatment of multiple nodular BCC's

[B] Involves the use of the photosensitizing drug 5-alphalevulinic acid to create free radicals

[C] Is a useful modality of treatment of actinic keratosis

[D] Is not suitable for the treatment of superficial BCC's

Q 1.18
Which of the following statements MOST accurately describes the histological appearance of a basal cell carcinoma?

[A] Irregular masses of squamous epithelium proliferating downwards into the dermis

[B] Presence of large eosinophilic cells

[C] Nests of small basophilic cells with a pattern of peripheral palisading

[D] Atypical keratinocytes with normal basal cells

Q 1.19
Excision of a 15 mm in diameter well-defined BCC with a 3mm peripheral margin is likely to clear in the tumour in what proportion of cases?

[A] 75%

[B] 85%

[C] 95%

[D] 98%

Q 1.20
A 45 year-old patient underwent an excision of a pigmented lesion on the left forearm. The histology report comes back as an almost completely regressed superficial spreading malignant melanoma and that it was impossible to estimate the Breslow thickness of the lesion. After discussing this case at the appropriate multi-disciplinary meeting, what is the most appropriate line of management?

[A] Perform a wider excision of the biopsy scar to reduce the risk of local recurrence of the melanoma

[B] Perform a sentinel lymph node biopsy to increase the chance of survival

[C] Arrange a staging CT scan

[D] Do nothing more

Q 1.21
Which of the following bacteria can be transmitted by leeches?

[A] *Aeromonas hydrophilia*

[B] *Eikenella corrodens*

[C] *Pasturella multocida*

[D] *Streptococcus viridans*

Q 1.22
Which of the following nerves does not provide sensory innervation to the ear?

[A] The greater auricular nerve

[B] The lesser auricular nerve

[C] The auriculotemporal nerve

[D] The vagus nerve

Q 1.23
A 77 year-old man presents with a primary tumour of the right side of the oral cavity of 1.8cm in diameter. On further examination he was found to have multiple enlarged right cervical lymph nodes none larger than 2cm in diameter. A staging CT scan revealed no evidence of distant metastases. What is the appropriate stage of the disease?

[A] Stage 1

[B] Stage 2

[C] Stage 3

[D] Stage 4

Q 1.24
Which structure(s) are sacrificed in a Type 1 modified radical neck dissection?

[A] The accessory nerve

[B] The internal jugular vein

[C] The sternocleidomastoid muscle and internal jugular vein

[D] The sternocleidomastoid muscle and accessory nerve

Q 1.25
The contents of which of the following levels are removed in a supraomohyoid selective neck dissection?

[A] 1, 2, 3

[B] 2, 3, 4

[C] 1, 2, 3, 4

[D] 2, 3, 4, 5

Q 1.26
The scalp is well vascularised by a rich vascular plexus. Which of the following does NOT contribute to the blood supply of the scalp?

[A] The superficial temporal artery

[B] The supraorbital artery

[C] The middle meningeal artery

[D] The postauricular artery

Q 1.27
In carrying out an augmentation-mastopexy procedure which of the following incisions is never used?

[A] Vertical incision

[B] Inverted T-shaped incision

[C] Circumareolar incision

[D] None of the above

Q 1.28
Which of the following muscles does NOT contribute to forming the posterior wall of the axilla?

[A] Latissimus dorsi

[B] Subscapularis

[C] Teres minor

[D] Teres major

Q 1.29
What is the mechanism of action of tamoxifen?

[A] It blocks oestrogen receptors in breast tissue

[B] It binds to oestrogen thus decreasing the serum concentration of oestrogen

[C] It blocks progesterone receptors in breast tissue

[D] It stimulates the action of oestrogen in breast tissue

Q 1.30
What is the MOST common cause of leg ulcers?

[A] Diabetic neuropathy

[B] Venous hypertension

[C] Squamous cell carcinoma

[D] Trauma

Q 1.31
What is the mechanism of action of 5-fluorouracil (Efudix®)?

[A] Deactivates cell membrane receptors

[B] Inhibits thymidylate synthase interfering with RNA and DNA synthesis

[C] Stimulates production of interferon alpha

[D] Inhibits the formation of interleukin-2

Q 1.32
Which of the statements regarding haemangiomas is FALSE?

[A] They are true neoplasms

[B] They are more common in females

[C] They occur most commonly in the perineal region

[D] They can occur at birth

Q 1.33
Which of the following statements most accurately describes the ideal position of the eyebrow in a woman?

[A] It lies 1mm above the superior orbital rim

[B] It lies level to the superior orbital rim

[C] The medial aspect of the eyebrow lies medial to a vertical perpendicular line through the alar base

[D] The medial and lateral ends of the eyebrow lie on the same horizontal level

Q 1.34
Which of the following statements most accurately describes the highest point of the female eyebrow?

[A] The junction of the medial and middle third

[B] Lies in the vertical plane of the lateral aspect of the corneal limbus

[C] Lies in the vertical plane of the medial aspect of the limbus

[D] Lies at the level of the superior orbital rim

Q 1.35
Which of the following is NOT a feature of the aging ear?

[A] A lesser conchoscaphoid angle

[B] An overall increase in the height of the ear

[C] An increase in the size of the earlobe

[D] An increase in the prominence of the ear

Q 1.36
Which of the following is a feature of the aging nose?

[A] Narrowing of the nostrils

[B] Enlargement and thickening of the alar cartilages

[C] An increase in the nasolabial angle

[D] Thinning of the overlying skin envelope

Q 1.37
A patient with premature aging secondary to which of the following conditions is likely to benefit from a facelift?

[A] Ehlers-Danlos syndrome

[B] Progeria

[C] Cutis laxa

[D] Werner's syndrome

Q 1.38
Which ONE of the following statements is FALSE?

[A] Clinically apparent photodamage is related to skin type

[B] Fair-skinned individuals are less likely to be susceptible to photodamage

[C] Broad spectrum sunscreens can protect against photoaging

[D] Photoaging increases with UV exposure

Q 1.39
Which one of the following is NOT a clinical feature of photoaging?

[A] Increased skin thickness

[B] Purpura

[C] Telangiectasia

[D] Coarse wrinkles

Q 1.40
Which of the following cell types has a mesodermal origin?

[A] Keratinocytes

[B] Merkel cells

[C] Langerhan's cells

[D] Melanocytes

QUIZ 1

EXTENDED MATCHING QUESTIONS

For questions 1.41 to 1.45 please select the ONE MOST appropriate answer from list [A] to [K]. Each answer maybe used more than once or not at all.

A Z-plasty is used to correct a linear, discreet, contracted scar across the volar aspect of the proximal interphalangeal joint of the right hand. The following figures represent possible theoretical gain in length of the scar.

[A] 10%
[B] 20%
[C] 25%
[D] 30%
[E] 45%
[F] 50%
[G] 60%
[H] 75%
[J] 100%
[K] 125%

What would be the theoretical gain in length obtained in the above case for the following angles of z-plasty:

1.41 30^0
1.42 45^0
1.43 60^0
1.44 75^0
1.45 90^0

For questions 1.46 to 1.50 please select the ONE MOST appropriate answer from list [A] to [K]. Each answer maybe used more than once or not at all.

The following is a list of skin malignancies.

[A] Basal cell carcinoma
[B] Squamous cell carcinoma
[C] Lentigo maligna
[D] Malignant melanoma
[E] Extramammary Paget disease
[F] Merkel cell carcinoma
[G] Trichilemmal carcinoma
[H] Atypical fibroxanthoma
[J] Dermatofibrosarcoma protuberans
[K] Microcystic adnexal carcinoma

Which one of the skin malignancies listed above best fits with the description below.

1.46 This is not treated by Moh's surgery?

1.47 May develop from an area of chronic inflammation and scarring?

1.48 Arises from the pluripotential cells of the basal layer of the epidermis?

1.49 A very aggressive type of skin malignancy which is very sensitive to radiotherapy?

1.50 Arises from keratinocytes of the stratum spinosum of the epidermis?

QUIZ 1
ANSWERS

1.1
Answer C
This wound has healed by secondary intention resulting in an extended contracted scar. The dermal elements of the skin would be absent. Hence, this would result in a decrease or absence of thermoregulation and sensation. Scars have a diminished protective function against ultraviolet light and hence patients should be advised of sun-protective measures.

1.2
Answer A
The stratum lucidum also known as the clear layer is only present in the thickened glaborous skin of the palms and soles of feet.

1.3
Answer B
The epidermis contains keratinocytes, Langerhan's cells, Merkel cells and melanocytes. Fibroblasts produce collagen, elastin and glycosaminoglycans (GAG's) which are all components of the dermis.

1.4
Answer B
Thromboxanes stimulate the conversion of fibrinogen to fibrin resulting in the propagation of the thrombus in the haemostatic phase of wound healing.

1.5
Answer A
In the remodelling phase of wound healing there is an involution of the capillary network in the scar. The rate of collagen production matches that of collagen degradation. The collagen fibres are arranged in a more orderly fashion and the 5:1 ratio of type 1 to type 3 collagen is restored.

1.6
Answer B
Prolongation of the inflammatory phase of wound healing has been implicated in the formation of hypertrophic scars.

1.7
Answer B
The characteristics of laser light are:
- Monochromatic
- Collimated
- Coherent

It selectively targets a specific chromophore in its mode of action (selective photothermolysis).

1.8
Answer C
Seventy percent of the expanded skin is due to stretch and 30% to new cells and growth. Expanded skin has an improved blood supply compared to the normal surrounding skin.

1.9
Answer C
Tessier cleft no. 7 is the most common type of craniofacial cleft. It originates at the commissure of the lip and extends laterally towards the ear.

1.10
Answer D
The metopic suture is the first cranial suture to fuse. This occurs at 2 years of age.

1.11
Answer D
Allografts refer to non-living tissue derived from the same species eg. Cadaveric skin.

1.12
Answer C
The primary palate consists of the lip, alveolus and the hard palate anterior to the incisive foramen. It is due to failure of fusion of the medial nasal process and the maxillary process.

1.13
Answer D
The overall incidence of cleft lip and palate is 1 in 1000 live birth. In Asia it is 1 in 500 live births and in Africa it is about 1 in 2000 live births.

1.14
Answer D
Giant congenital hairy naevii are not confined to the dermis and may invade underlying structures. There is a 5 – 10% risk of malignant transformation.

1.15
Answer C
The cardinal signs of a sarcoma are;
- Size >5cm
- Associated pain
- Deep to fascia
- Increasing in size
  The likelihood of a soft tissue sarcoma with all 4 cardinal signs is 86%.

1.16
Answer C
Gorlins syndrome is an autosomal dominant condition which is associated with multiple BCCs occurring at a young age. Other features includes large head, bifid ribs, odontogenic keratocysts, cardiac and ovarian fibromas, shortened 4th metacarpals and palmar pits.

1.17
Answer C
Photodynamic therapy involves the use of the photosensitizing drug 5-aminolevulinic acid to create free radicals that destroys target cells. Is a useful modality of treatment of actinic keratosis and superficial BCC's.

1.18
Answer C
The histological appearance of a basal cell carcinoma involves the presence of sheets or nests of small, round basophilic cells which demonstrate peripheral pallisading.

1.19
Answer B
Excision of a well-defined BCC with a diameter of <20mm with a 3mm peripheral margin is likely to clear in the tumour in 85% of cases. A 4mm peripheral margin in such cases is likely to clear the tumour in 95% of cases. In morphoeic and larger BCC's a 13 – 15mm peripheral margin is required to clear the tumour in 95% of cases.

1.20
Answer A
Although a Breslow thickness cannot be estimated, this represents a regressed invasive malignant melanoma and hence a wider excision of the previous biopsy scar is warranted to minimise the risk of local recurrence.

1.21
Answer A
Patients having leech therapy should be prophylactic antibiotics against *Aeromonas hydrophilia*.

1.22
Answer B
The greater auricular nerve innervates the lower half of the external ear. The auriculotemporal nerve innervates the lateral aspect of the upper half of the ear and a branch of the vagus nerve contributes to the innervations of the external auditory meatus.

1.23
Answer D
This presentation is a T1 N2b M0 which makes it stage 4 disease.

1.24
Answer C
The following structures are **preserved** in modified radical neck dissection
Type 1: The accessory nerve
Type 2: The accessory nerve and the sternocleidomastoid muscle
Type 3: The accessory nerve, the sternocleidomastoid muscle and the internal jugular vein

1.25
Answer A
In a supraomohyoid selective neck dissection the contents of the levels 1, 2 and 3 are removed.

1.26
Answer C
The scalp is richly vascularised by a plexus formed by the superficial temporal, posterior auricular and occipital branches of the external carotid and by the supraorbital and supratrochlear branches of the internal carotid artery. The middle meningeal artery is a branch of the maxillary artery (external carotid). It passes underneath the pterion and supplies the meninges.

1.27
Answer D
Although it usually involves a vertical skin incision, inverted T incisions as well as cicumareolar incisions maybe used.

1.28
Answer C
The axilla is formed by the following structures:
Anterior wall: Pectoralis major and minor, subclavius
Posterior wall: Latissimus dorsi, subscapularis and teres major
Lateral wall: Coracobrachialis and biceps
Medial wall: Chest wall comprising upper 5 ribs, intercostals and serratus anterior

1.29
Answer A
Tamoxifen is a selective oestrogen receptor modulator which works by blocking the oestrogen receptors in breast tissue.

1.30
Answer B
Venous hypertension is the most cause of leg ulceration.

1.31
Answer B
5-fluorouracil is an anti-metabolite. It inhibits thymidylate synthase which is an enzyme involved in nucleotide metabolism.

1.32
Answer C
Most haemangiomas occur in the head and neck region (60%). They are true neoplasms of the endothelial cells. They are 3 times more common in female infants. Although most haemangiomas are not present at birth and appear soon afterwards, there is an entity known as congenital haemangiomas which are present at birth.

1.33
Answer D
The position of the ideal eyebrow of a female lies approximately 1cm above the superior orbital rim whereas, in males it lies at the level of the superior orbital rim. The medial end of the eyebrow falls in a vertical perpendicular line through the alar base. The medial and lateral ends of the female eyebrow lie on the same horizontal level.

1.34
Answer B
The highest point of the female eyebrow lies in the vertical plane of the lateral aspect of the corneal limbus.

1.35
Answer A
There is an overall prominence of the aging ear because of an increase in the conchoscaphoid angle and an increase in the vertical height due to an increase in the size of the earlobe.

1.36
Answer B
The features of the aging nose are:
- Widening of the nostrils
- Enlargement and thickening of the alar cartilages
- A decrease in the nasolabial angle
- Thickening of the overlying skin

1.37
Answer C
Aesthetic surgery is contraindicated in patients with Ehlers-Danlos syndrome, Progeria and Werner's syndrome.

1.38
Answer B
Clinically apparent photodamage is related to skin type, with fair-skinned being more susceptible.

1.39
Answer A
With photoaging, skin becomes thinner. The clinical features of photoaging are: Fine and coarse wrinkles, skin laxity, purpura, telangiectasia, irregular pigmentation and fat redistribution.

1.40
Answer C
Keratinocytes form the major cell type in the epidermis and are derived from ectoderm. Merkel cells and melanocytes have a neural crest origin. Langerhan's cells are derived from precursor cells of the bone marrow (mesodermal origin).

1.41
ANSWER C

1.42
ANSWER F

1.43
ANSWER H

1.44
ANSWER J

1.45
ANSWER K

1.46
ANSWER D

1.47
ANSWER B

**1.48
ANSWER A**

**1.49
ANSWER F**

**1.50
ANSWER B**

QUIZ 2
MULTIPLE CHOICE QUESTIONS

For questions 2.1 to 2.40 please the ONE most appropriate answer.

Q 2.1
Which ONE of the following types of laser is most suitable for the treatment of port-wine stains?

[A] Pulse dye lasers

[B] Q-switched KTP lasers

[C] Diode lasers

[D] Nd:YAG lasers

Q 2.2
Which ONE of the following techniques is NOT useful in periorbital rejuvenation?

[A] Blepharoplasty

[B] Radiotherapy

[C] Botulinum toxin

[D] Chemical peels

Q 2.3
The Asian upper eyelid is different from the Caucasian upper eyelid in the all of the following ways EXCEPT?

[A] The eyelid crease is lower

[B] There is the presence of preaponeurotic fat anterior to the tarsus

[C] Mullers muscles are absent

[D] The orbital septum fuses with the levator aponeurosis more distally

Q 2.4
A 27 year-old gentleman presents with a pulsatile lump in the region of the thenar eminence of his dominant right hand which has features of a vascular malformation. What is the most appropriate mode of treatment of this lesion?

[A] Systemic steroids

[B] Intralesional steroid injection

[C] Angiography and ligation of the feeding vessel

[D] Angiography and embolisation of the nidus of the AVM, followed by surgical excision and reconstruction.

Q 2.5
Which of the following is the main advantage of using the pectoralis minor muscle as opposed to the gracilis for facial reanimation?

[A] The donor site is more easily accessible

[B] The donor scarring is more acceptable

[C] The pectoralis minor muscle has a higher density of neuromuscular units

[D] The vascular pedicle of the pectoralis muscle is more suitable for microsurgical transfer

Q 2.6
Which one of the following is the MOST favourable incision for a lip-split/mandibulotomy for access to a adenocystic carcinoma confined to the left side of the soft palate?

[A] |

[B] ⊃

[C] Ć

[D] ᴗ

Q 2.7
What is the mechanism of action of Botulinum toxin?

[A] It stimulates the production of collagen which is incorporated into the tissues

[B] It activates mechanisms to rearrange the dermal collagen in a more orderly fashion

[C] It blocks the post-synaptic action of acetylcholine at the neuro-muscular junction

[D] It blocks the pre-synaptic action of acetylcholine at the neuro-muscular junction at a site proximal to the release of the acetylcholine

Q 2.8
Which of the following most closely matches the incidence of hypospadias?

[A] 1:30 live male births

[B] 1:300 live male births

[C] 1:3000 live male births

[D] 1:30000 live male births

Q 2.9
In cases of lower limb trauma, muscle flaps have a distinct advantage over fasciocutaneous flaps in which of the following way?

[A] They heal better

[B] They conform better to the defect

[C] Reoperations are better facilitated by the ease of flap elevation to provide bony access

[D] The cosmetic outcome is generally better

Q 2.10
Which of the following is NOT a feature of tuberous breast deformity?

[A] A narrow base of breast

[B] Herniation of breast tissue through the nipple-areolar complex

[C] A superiorly displaced inframammary fold

[D] Hypoplasia of muscles of the anterior chest wall

Q .2.11
A 21 year-old woman presents with a right sided tuberous breast deformity which involves a constricted base with hyploplasia of the medial and lateral lower quadrants with sufficient subareolar skin. Using the classification described by von Heimburg et al, this is a description of which type of tuberous breast deformity?

[A] Type I

[B] Type II

[C] Type III

[D] Type IV

35

Q 2.12
With regards to gynaecomastia which of the following statements is TRUE?

[A] Gynaecomastia always occurs bilaterally

[B] Gynaecomastia is bilateral in about a half of cases

[C] Gynaecomastia occurs on the left side more commonly

[D] Gynaecomastia is rare in elderly men

Q 2.13
The lobule of the external ear is a derivative of which of the following embryological structures?

[A] Branchial arch I

[B] Branchial cleft I

[C] Branchial arch II

[D] Branchial cleft II

Q 2.14
Which of the following fascial layers surround the platysma muscle?

[A] The superficial cervical fascia

[B] The investing cervical fascia

[C] The pretracheal cervical fascia

[D] The prevertebral cervical fascia

Q 2.15
Which of the following statements most accurately describes the course of the spinal accessory nerve as it courses through the neck?

[A] It crosses the sternocleidomastoid muscle in the upper-middle third towards the middle-lower third of the trapezius

[B] It crosses the sternocleidomastoid muscle in the middle-lower third towards the middle-lower third of the trapezius

[C] It crosses the sternocleidomastoid muscle in the upper-middle third towards the upper-middle third of the trapezius

[D] It crosses the sternocleidomastoid muscle in the middle-lower third towards the upper-middle third of the trapezius

Q 2.16
Which of the following reconstructive techniques for the lower lip preserves motor and sensory functions?

[A] Abbe flap

[B] Eastlander flap

[C] Karapandzic flap

[D] Bernard flap

Q 2.17
Which of the following is NOT a suitable mode of reconstruction of the upper lip in a patient who would like to wear a moustache?
[A] McGregor flap

[B] Islanded pedicled temporal scalp flap based on the superficial temporal artery

[C] Washio flap

[D] Pedicled nasolabial flap

37

Q 2.18
Which of the following vessels does NOT contribute to the blood supply of the sternocleidomastoid muscle?

[A] Superior thyroid artery

[B] Occipital artery

[C] Thyrocervical trunk

[D] Facial artery

Q 2.19
In reconstructing a full-thickness defect of the nose which of the following is the most important layer to consider?

[A] Inner lining

[B] Cartilaginous structures

[C] Muscle layer

[D] Outer layer (skin)

Q 2.20
What is the MOST appropriate technique for the reconstruction of the entire eyebrow in a patient who underwent radiotherapy of that area?

[A] Micrograft hair follicle transplantation

[B] Hair strip grafts

[C] Pedicled postauricular temporoparietal scalp flap

[D] Scalp rotation flap

Q 2.21
What is the anatomical basis for the difference between the Asian and Caucasian upper eyelids?

[A] Predominantly greater density of dermal attachments of the levator aponeurosis

[B] Lack of dermal attachments of the fibres of the levator aponeurosis

[C] The orbital septum is attached to the levator aponeurosis at a higher point

[D] A relative lack of preaponeurotic fat

Q 2.22
A 77 year-old man presents with a primary tumour of the right side of the oral cavity of 1.8cm in diameter. On further examination he was found to have multiple enlarged right cervical lymph nodes none larger than 2cm in diameter. An FNA has confirmed nodal metastases. A staging CT scan revealed no evidence of distant metastases. The patient is otherwise medically fit. You plan to excise the primary tumour. What would be your management of the neck?

[A] Open excision biopsy of one of the nodes

[B] A radical neck dissection

[C] A modified radical neck dissection Type 2

[D] A supraomohyoid neck dissection to reduce post-op morbidity

Q 2.23
Using the Tanzer classification of ear deformities, which of the following types would cryptotia fall under?
[A] Type 1

[B] Type 4A

[C] Type 4B

[D] Type 4C

Q 2.24
Three hours after performing a free groin flap to reconstruct a defect on the dorsum of the left hand, it is observed that the flap has become pale, feels cool and a capillary refill time cannot be established. The room is warm and the patient is well hydrated. What is your next step in the management of this patient?

[A] Assume that there a thrombosis of the venous anastomosis and fully anticoagulate the patient

[B] Assume that there is a thrombosis of the venous anastomosis and return the patient to Theatre

[C] Assume that there is a thrombosis of the arterial anastomosis, take down to dressings to relieve any potential constricting effect and make arrangements to return the patient to theatre without delay

[D] Since this is a new clinical change in the status of the flap, it should be reviewed over next few hours to monitor the development prior to making a definitive decision

Q 2.25
A 43 year-old gentleman presents with a 6-month history of a 10cm in diameter lesion on the anterior aspect of the left thigh. After clinically evaluating this patient in the clinic what would you do next?

[A] Attempt to perform a fine needle biopsy of the lesion in the clinic

[B] Attempt to obtain a core biopsy in the clinic

[C] Request an MRI scan of the area prior to performing a core biopsy

[D] Request an ultrasound scan of the lesion

Q 2.26
Which of the following is the most common type of BCC?

[A] Superficial

[B] Nodular

[C] Pigmented

[D] Morpheic

Q 2.27
Which of the following is NOT a recognised feature of Gorlin's syndrome?

[A] It has an autosomal recessive pattern of inheritance

[B] Always presents with a history of multiple BCC's

[C] Can present with bifid ribs

[D] Patients with Gorlin's syndrome may have learning difficulties

Q 2.28
A primary SCC occurring in which of the following sites has the WORST prognosis (assuming that all other factors are constant)?

[A] Lower leg

[B] Penis

[C] Lower lip

[D] A chronic ulcer

Q 2.29
A 35 year-old gentleman presents to the Outpatient Clinic for wider excision of the scar of a 2.5mm Breslow thickness non-ulcerated malignant melanoma from his upper back. He must undergo which of the following investigations?

[A] A baseline chest x-ray and abdominal ultrasound

[B] A baseline CT scan of the abdomen

[C] A staging CT scan of the chest, abdomen and pelvis

[D] None of the above

Q 2.30
What is the MOST common type of malignant melanoma in Caucasians?

[A] Superficial spreading melanoma

[B] Nodular melanoma

[C] Lentigo maligna melanoma

[D] Acral lentiginous melanoma

Q 2.31
Which of the following techniques used in repairing a relatively large palatal fistula is MOST likely to result in a recurrence of the fistula?

[A] Use of a cartilage graft

[B] Repair of the fistula by mobilising the palatal mucosa

[C] Repair of the fistula using a vomerine flap and a pedicled cheek mucosal transposition flap

[D] Using a bone graft

Q 2.32
Which of the following is NOT a feature of DiGeorge syndrome?

[A] Hypocalcaemia

[B] Cleft palate

[C] A long face with prominent epicanthic folds

[D] Hypothyroidism

Q 2.33
Which of the following is NOT a source of autogenous cartilage?

[A] Soft palate

[B] Nasal septum

[C] Pinna

[D] Rib

Q 2.34
Which of the following is a result of a metopic synostosis?

[A] Plagiocephaly

[B] Scaphocephaly

[C] Trigonocephaly

[D] Brachycephaly

Q 2.35
Which of the following is a characteristic feature of Mobius syndrome?

[A] Bilateral facial atrophy

[B] Bilateral involvement of the cranial nerves VII only

[C] Bilateral involvement of the cranial nerves VI and VII

[D] It is associated with mental underdevelopment

Q 2.36
In expanded tissue all of the following structures thin out EXCEPT?

[A] The epidermis

[B] The dermis

[C] The subcutaneous tissue

[D] Muscle

Q 2.37
What is the wavelength range for ultraviolet light?

[A] 200 – 400nm

[B] 400 – 755nm

[C] 755 – 1400nm

[D] 1400 – 2800nm

Q 2.38
Which isoform of TGF-β has been shown to decrease scarring?

[A] TGF-β Type 1

[B] TGF-β Type 2

[C] TGF-β Type 3

[D] TGF-β Type 4

Q 2.39
Which of the following statements about Ehlers-Danlos syndrome is FALSE?

[A] It involves a defect in the synthesis and processing of collagen

[B] Can present with hypermobile fingers

[C] It is safe to carry out elective aesthetic procedures on these patients

[D] Can present with hyperextensible skin

Q 2.40
Smoking has all of the following effects on tissue perfusion EXCEPT?

[A] The increased levels of carbon dioxide in the smoke shifts the oxygen dissociation curve to the left resulting in decreased tissue oxygenation

[B] The increased levels of carbon monoxide in the smoke shifts the oxygen dissociation curve to the left resulting in decreased tissue oxygenation

[C] Nicotine in the smoke results in vasoconstriction

[D] Decreased tissue perfusion

QUIZ 2
EXTENDED MATCHING QUESTIONS

For questions 2.41 to 2.45 please select the ONE MOST appropriate answer from list [A] to [K]. Each answer maybe used more than once or not at all.

QUESTION x

The following is a list of congenital abnormalities of the hand.

[A] Syndactyly

[B] Symphalangism

[C] Brachydactyly

[D] Polydactyly

[E] Camptodactyly

[F] Clinodactyly

[G] Radial club hand

[H] Ulnar club hand

[J] Arthrogryposis

[K] Macrodactyly

Which one of the options listed above best fit each of the descriptions outlined below?

Q 2.41
Results from a congenital overgrowth defect?

Q 2.42
Maybe associated with Fanconi's anaemia?

Q 2.43
A condition thought to arise from failure of apoptosis within the interdigital tissues during embryonic development and maybe associated with Apert's syndrome?

Q 2.44
A congenital deformity characterised by a flexion deformity of the proximal interphalangeal joint most commonly affecting the little finger?

Q 2.45
A congenital condition which presents with bilateral contractures of the elbow and adduction and internal rotation of the shoulders?

For questions 2.46 to 2.50 please select the ONE MOST appropriate answer from list [A] to [K]. Each answer maybe used more than once or not at all.

The following is a list of various classifications of flaps.

[A] Mathes and Nahai Type I

[B] Mathes and Nahai Type II

[C] Mathes and Nahai Type III

[D] Mathes and Nahai Type IV

[E] Mathes and Nahai Type V

[F] Random-pattern flap

[G] Axial-pattern flap

[H] Perforator flap

[J]   Interpositional flap

[K] Free flap

Which are the flaps outlined below best classified?

Q 2.46 Latissimus dorsi muscle flap

Q 2.47 A serratus muscle flap used to reconstruct a defect of the leg following a crush injury to the leg

Q 2.48 A rectus abdominis muscle flap

Q 2.49 Triple-rhomboid flaps to reconstruct a defect on the back

Q 2.50 Gracilis muscle flap

QUIZ 2
ANSWERS

2.1
Answer A
Pulse dye lasers are considered the treatment of choice for port-wine stains and spider angiomas.

2.2
Answer B
The techniques that are useful in periorbital rejuvenation are blepharoplasty, botulinum toxin, fillers, chemical peels, ablative resurfacing, fractionated skin resurfacing.

2.3
Answer C
The Asian upper eyelid is different from that of Caucasians in that the orbital septum fuses with the levator aponeurosis more distally, there is preaponeurotic fat anterior to the tarsus and the eyelid crease is lower.

2.4
Answer D
This fits the description of an arteriovenous malformation. It is best treated by embolisation into the nidus of the lesion and followed by surgical excision within 24 – 72 hours. Simply ligating the feeding vessel is contraindication since it results in an increase in the number of collateral vessels and the size of the lesion.

2.5
Answer C
The pectoralis muscle has a higher density of neuromuscular junctions than the gracilis muscle. Hence, it is known as the 'smart' muscle.

2.6
Answer B
A curved-shaped incision around the lateral margin of the chin towards the side of the lesion is desirable.

2.7
Answer D
Botulinum toxin works by blocking the pre-synaptic action of acetylcholine at the neuro-muscular junction at a site proximal to the release of the acetylcholine by disrupting the calcium-mediated release of the neuro-transmitter, acetylcholine.

2.8
Answer B
The incidence of hypospadias is 1:300 live male births.

2.9
Answer B
Muscle flaps conform to defects better than the less pliable fasciocutaneous flaps. They donot however heal better than fasciocutaneous flaps. In general fasciocutaneous flaps are cosmetically superior and can provide easier bony access in cases of reoperations for bony reconstruction.

2.10
Answer D
Hypoplasia of the anterior chest wall is a feature of Poland's syndrome and not tuberous breast deformity. The features of tuberous breast deformity are;
- A constricted breast base
- A thin elongated breast
- Widened areolar
- Herniation of the breast parenchyma through the nipple areolar complex
- Superior displacement of the inframammary fold

2.11
Answer B
The von Heimburg classification of tuberous breast deformity:
Type I: Hypoplasia of the lower medial quadrant
Type II: Hypoplasia of the lower medial and lateral quadrants with sufficient subareolar skin
Type III: Hypoplasia of the lower medial and lateral quadrants with a deficiency of subareolar skin
Type IV: Severe base of breast constriction

2.12
Answer B
Gynaecomastia occurs bilaterally in about 50% – 55% of cases. In unilateral cases, it more commonly occurs on the right side. There is an increased incidence in elderly men.

2.13
Answer C
The antihelix, antitragus and lobule of the external ear are all derivatives of the second branchial arch.

2.14
Answer A
The platysma is a discrete muscle of the panniculus carnosus. Although it is a discrete striated muscle it is part of the subcutaneous tissues of the neck lying deep to the panniculus adiposus.

2.15
Answer A
The spinal accessory nerve crosses the sternocleidomastoid muscle in the upper-middle third towards the middle-lower third of the trapezius 5cm above the clavicle. It is particularly prone to damage in cervical block dissections.

2.16
Answer C
In creating the Karapandzic flap the neurovascular structures are preserved by careful dissection.

2.17
Answer A
The McGregor flap is an advancement flap to reconstruct lower eyelid defects. It utilises a Z-plasty at the lateral end to encourage the flap to advance medially. The Washio (retroauricular-temporal) flap may be used to include hair-bearing tissue from the mastoid area.

2.18
Answer D
The blood supply to the sternocleidomastoid muscle is as follows:
Proximal third: Occipital artery
Middle third: Superior thyroid artery
Distal third: Branch of the thyrocervical trunk

2.19
Answer A
The inner lining is the most important. It should be thin to prevent nasal obstruction, it should conform to the shape of the nose and should be well-vascularised to support cartilage grafts.

2.20
Answer C
In a poorly vascularised recipient bed, it would unsuitable to use micrograft hair transplantation or hair strip grafts. The most appropriate option would be a pedicled postauricular temporoparietal scalp flap based on the superficial temporal artery.

2.21
Answer B
In the Asian upper eyelid there is a lack of dermal attachments of the fibres of the levator aponeurosis. This leads to the less prominent appearance of the supratarsal crease. The orbital septum has a lower attachment to the levator aponeurosis.

2.22
Answer B
This patient has N2b disease and therefore a radical neck dissection is warranted.

2.23
Answer C
The Tanzer classification of ear deformities:
- Type 1:   Anotia
- Type 2A: Microtia with atresia of the external auditory meatus
- Type 2B: Microtia without atresia of the external auditory meatus
- Type 3:   Hypoplasia of the middle-third of the ear
- Type 4A: Constricted ear
- Type 4B: Cryptotia
- Type 4C: Cryptotia of the upper third of the ear
- Type 5:   Prominent ear

2.24
Answer C
This flap is has no arterial input therefore points of potential constriction should be relieved and the patient should be returned to theatre for exploration of the arterial anastomosis. There should be no delay in instituting the above actions.

53

2.25
Answer C
Imaging should be performed prior to obtaining a core biopsy to avoid the potential distortion of the soft tissues by haemorrhage or oedema.

2.26
Answer B
Nodular BCCs is the most common subtype.

2.27
Answer A
Gorlin's syndrome has an autosomal dominant pattern of inheritance. It is characterised by a history of multiple BCC's and can present with palmar pits, bifid ribs, calcification of the falx cerebri of the brain, learning difficulties, odontogenic cysts and overdevelopment of the supraorbital ridges.

2.28
Answer D
SCC's involving the following sites are listed in order of increasing metastatic potential:
- Sun-exposed sites excluding the lip and ear
- Lip
- Ear
- Non-sun exposed sites
- Marjolin's ulcer

2.29
Answer D
This patient has Stage IIA disease and does not need to undergo any baseline or staging investigations by imaging.

2.30
Answer A
Superficial spreading melanoma is the most common clinical and histological type (60%) compared to nodular melanoma (30%).

2.31
Answer B
Repair of the palatal fistula with a single layer tissue repair is the least desireable technique and is the method associated with the greatest risk of recurrence.

2.32
Answer D
DiGeorge syndrome, also known as velocardiofacial syndrome and CATCH 22 syndrome, can present with:
- Cardiac anoamlies
- A long face with prominent epicanthic folds
- Thymic aplasia
- Cleft palate
- Hypocalcaemia

2.33
Answer A
The soft palate is not composed of cartilage but mucosa and muscle and has a functional role in velopharyngeal closure.

2.34
Answer C
Metopic synostosis results in trigonocephaly.

2.35
Answer C
Mobius syndrome is a rare congenital neurological disorder characterised by the underdevelopment of cranial nerves VI and VII bilaterally. These patients characteristically have normal intelligence but an expressionless face.

2.36
Answer A
In expanded tissue the epidermis thickens but the dermis, subcutaneous fat and muscles thins. The expanded tissue has an improved blood supply.

2.37
Answer A
The wavelength of ultraviolet light is in the range of 200 – 400nm. Visible light: 400 – 755nm.

2.38
Answer C
TGF-β Types 1 and 2 has been shown to promote scarring whereas Type 3 has been shown to decrease. Clinical trials are currently in progress.

2.39
Answer C
Elective surgery should be avoided in patients with Ehlers-Danlos syndrome because these patients are prone to wound healing problems. The underlying defect in this condition is faulty collagen synthesis and processing.

2.40
Answer A
The increased levels of **carbon monoxide** in the smoke shifts the oxygen dissociation curve to the left resulting in decreased tissue oxygenation. Carbon dioxide on the other hand results ina rightward shift of the oxygen dissociation curve (resulting in haemoglobin having a reduced affinity for oxygen). Nicotine in cigarette smoke has a direct vasoconstrictive effect resulting in decreased tissue perfusion

2.41
Answer K

2.42
Answer G

2.43
Answer A

2.44
Answer E

2.45
Answer J

2.46
Answer E

2.47
Answer C

2.48
Answer C

2.49
Answer F

2.50
Answer B

QUIZ 3
MULTIPLE CHOICE QUESTIONS

For questions 3.1 to 3.40 please the ONE most appropriate answer.

Q 3.1

Which of the following statements most appropriately describes the function of Langerhan's cells?

[A] Function as antigen-presenting cells (APC's)

[B] Function as mechanoreceptors

[C] Provide protection by absorbing ultra-violet light

[D] Function as pressure receptors

Q 3.2

A 7year-old boy has developed a hypertrophic postauricular scar following prominent ear correction done 6 months ago. What is the likely ratio of the proportion of Type 1 collagen compared to Type 3 collagen within this scar?

[A] 5:1

[B] 1:5

[C] 1:6

[D] 2:1

Q 3.3

Which of the following results in an inhibition of hydroxylation of proline during collagen synthesis?

[A] Triamcinolone

[B] Colchicine

[C] A deficiency of vitamin C

[D] A deficiency of copper

Q 3.4
Macrophages are essential cells in the process of wound healing. Which of the following is NOT a recognised function of macrophages in wound healing?

[A] Act as phagocytes

[B] Attract fibroblasts

[C] Produce interleukin-3

[D] Coordinate the activity of fibroblasts through the production of TGF-β

Q 3.5
Fetal wound healing in the first trimester differs from normal wound healing in which of the following way?

[A] The inflammatory phase is prolonged

[B] Increased angiogenesis in the proliferative phase

[C] Has a decreased proportion of water

[D] Has a greater proportion of Type 3 collagen rather than Type 1

Q 3.6
Which of the following factors would adverse affect the survival of a non-vascularised bone graft?

[A] Bone graft with an intact periosteum

[B] A bone graft placed in an orthotopic position

[C] A bone graft placed in a heterotopic position

[D] A rigidly fixed bone graft

Q 3.7
A third-degree injury to a peripheral nerve according to the Sunderland classification of nerve injury corresponds to which one of the following statements?

[A] Axonal injury with preservation of all of its surrounding connective tissue sheaths

[B] Axonal injury with division of the endoneurium only

[C] Division of all intraneural structures but with preservation of the epineurium

[D] Complete division of the peripheral nerve

Q 3.8
What microbiological load is required to cause a clinical wound infection?

[A] 10^{10}

[B] 10^{2}

[C] 10^{5}

[D] 10^{6}

Q 3.9
With regards to split-thickness skin grafts, which of the following statements is TRUE?

[A] There is greater primary contraction than full-thickness skin grafts

[B] There is greater secondary contraction than full-thickness skin grafts

[C] Do not conform as well to defects like full-thickness skin grafts do

[D] Meshing does not increase the surface area of the graft

Q 3.10
Which of the following is NOT a characteristic of laser energy?

[A] It can be absorbed

[B] It can be reflected

[C] It can be transmitted through a medium

[D] It does not scatter

Q 3.11
Which of the following best describes the mechanism of intraoperative expansion during the insertion of a breast expander for tubular breast deformity?

[A] Mechanical creep

[B] Biological creep

[C] Stress relaxation

[D] Plastic deformation

Q 3.12
Which of the following is not a feature of Goldenhar's syndrome?

[A] Hemifacial microsomia

[B] Autosomal dominant inheritance

[C] Epibulbar dermoids

[D] Vertebral abnormailities

Q 3.13
Which of the following statements is TRUE of Alloderm®?

[A] It is derived from the skin of pigs

[B] It is a permanent skin substitute

[C] It is highly allergenic

[D] It is acellular human cadaveric dermis

Q 3.14
Which is the MOST common form of cleft lip?

[A] Right unilateral cleft lip

[B] Left unilateral cleft lip

[C] Isolated cleft lip

[D] Bilateral cleft lip

Q 3.15
A 15 year old boy has an isolated left unilateral cleft lip repaired in infancy. On further examination he has multiple pits of the lower lip and an absence of the second premolar tooth on the left side. His intellectual development is normal. What is the MOST likely diagnosis?

[A] Apert's syndrome

[B] Goldenhar's syndrome

[C] Van der Woude syndrome

[D] Treacher Collins syndrome

Q 3.16
What is the main functional muscle of the soft palate producing velopharyngeal closure?

[A] Tensor veli palatini

[B] Levator veli palatine

[C] Muscularis uvulae

[D] Stylopharyngeus

Q 3.17
Which nerve innervates the tensor veli palatini muscle?

[A] CN V

[B] CN VII

[C] CN IX

[D] CN X

Q 3.18
Which of the types of primary skin cancer has the worst prognosis?

[A] Basal cell carcinoma

[B] Squamous cell carcinoma

[C] Merkel cell carcinoma

[D] Malignant melanoma

Q 3.19
A patient with Fitzpatrick Type I skin on exposure to sunlight?

[A] Always burns, never tans

[B] Usually burns

[C] Always tans, never burns

[D] Rarely burns

Q 3.20
A morphoeic BCC is classified as a/an?

[A] Localised BCC

[B] Infiltrative BCC

[C] Superficial BCC

[D] Micronodular BCC

Q 3.21
What is the 5-year survival rate following metastatic SCC?

[A] 7%

[B] 15%

[C] 35%

[D] 65%

Q 3.22
Which of the following statements MOST accurately describes 'marginal excision' of a soft tissue sarcoma?

[A] The plane of excision extends into the lesion

[B] The plane of excision runs through the pseudocapsule surrounding the tumour

[C] The plane of excision extends into the normal surrounding tissues but is within the same compartment as the tumour

[D] The tumour and the contents of the compartment are excised together

Q 3.23
Which of the following substances is secreted by leeches?

[A] Antithrombin III

[B] Prostaglandin

[C] Heparan sulphate

[D] Hirudin

Q 3.24
What is the most common cause of surface irregularity of the external ear?

[A] Costochondritis

[B] Post-surgical

[C] Congenital deformity

[D] Trauma

Q 3.25
Which of the following statements regarding salivary gland tumours is FALSE?

[A] Salivary gland tumours account for about 20% of all head and neck malignancies

[B] Most salivary gland tumours occur in the parotid gland

[C] Most parotid gland tumours are benign

[D] The most common parotid gland tumour is pleomorphic adenoma

Q 3.26
Which of the following statements regarding Warthin's tumour is FALSE?

[A] Commonly found in the tail of the parotid gland

[B] 10% are bilateral

[C] Is a malignant tumour of the parotid gland

[D] Treated by superficial parotidectomy

Q 3.27
Which of the following is NOT an indication for an open biopsy of neck lump?

[A] Suspected metastasis from a previously excised preauricular SCC

[B] Following a negative FNA of the lump

[C] Suspected lymphoma

[D] Unable to establish a diagnosis following a negative FNA and negative panendoscopy with multiple random biopsies

Q 3.28
Which of the following fascial layers surround the parotid gland?

[A] The superficial cervical fascia

[B] The investing cervical fascia

[C] The pretracheal cervical fascia

[D] The prevertebral cervical fascia

Q 3.29
Which of the following is a landmark for the location of the facial nerve as it exits the stylomastoid foramen?

[A] It is superficial to the sternomastoid muscle

[B] It is lateral to the styloid process

[C] It is posterior to the posterior belly of the digastrics muscle

[D] It is anterior to the facial vein

Q 3.30
Which of the following is of ectodermal origin?

[A] Neural crest cells

[B] Bone

[C] Connective tissue

[D] Cartilage

Q 3.31
Which of the following vessels does NOT provide a blood supply to the breast

[A] Thoracoacromial artery

[B] Thyrocervical trunk

[C] Thoracodorsal artery

[D] Lateral thoracic artery

Q 3.32
What is the incidence of occult malignancies in breast reduction tissues?

[A] 1%

[B] 0.06%

[C] 0.6%

[D] 2%

Q 3.33
Using the Regnault classification of breast ptosis which of the following MOST closely describes a third degree breast ptosis?

[A] The nipple lies at the level of the inframammary fold (IMF) but the major portion of the breast tissue lies below the IMF

[B] The nipple and the most dependent portion of the breast lies below the inframammary fold

[C] The nipple lies below the inframammary fold but above the most dependent portion of the breast

[D] The nipple lies above the inframammary fold

Q 3.34
Which of the following statements regarding augmentation-mastopexy is CORRECT?

[A] It is generally easy to perform

[B] Minimises the risk of a double-bubble deformity in suitable patients

[C] It should always be done in two stages

[D] Is not suitable for the correction of third degree breast ptosis

Q 3.35
Which of the following is NOT a parameter for consideration when using the mangled extremity score?

[A] Co-morbidities

[B] Age of the patient

[C] Presence of shock

[D] Presence of pulses and sensation

Q 3.36
An increased distance between the medial walls of the orbit is known as?

[A] Telecanthus

[B] Hypertelorism

[C] Pseudotelecanthus

[D] Harlequin deformity

Q 3.37
What is the most common cause of ptosis?

[A] Congenital

[B] Myasthenia gravis

[C] Horner's syndrome

[D] Senile ptosis

Q 3.38
The wavelength of ultraviolet light in terrestrial sunlight is most likely to be?

[A] 290-400nm

[B] 400-700nm

[C] 700-850nm

[D] More than 900nm

Q 3.39
Which ONE of the following is most likely to cause photoaging?

[A] UVA

[B] UVB

[C] UVC

[D] Visible light

Q 3.40
Which of the following structures can be found to have the most yellow colour intra-operatively during upper lid blepharoplasty?

[A] The lacrimal gland

[B] The medial fat pad

[C] The middle fat pad

[D] The levator aponeurosis

QUIZ 3
EXTENDED MATCHING QUESTIONS

For questions 3.41 to 3.45 please select the ONE MOST appropriate answer from list [A] to [K]. Each answer maybe used more than once or not at all.

The following is list of biomaterials used as implant materials.

[A] Titanium
[B] Hydroxyapatite
[C] Bioactive glass
[D] Silicone
[E] Polyesters
[F] Polytetrafluoroethylene
[G] Polypropylene
[H] Collagen
[J] Gold
[K] Polyglycolic acid

Which of the following does the descriptions below best fit?

Q 3.41 Biodegadable polyester?

Q 3.42 A corrosive-resistant metal with poor strength?

Q 3.43 A calcium ceramic?

Q 3.44 A non-absorbable suture material?

Q 3.45 A biologic material?

For questions 3.46 to 3.50 please select the ONE MOST appropriate answer from list [A] to [K]. Each answer maybe used more than once or not at all.

With regards to nerve injuries.

[A] First degree

[B] Second degree

[C] Third degree

[D] Fourth Degree

[E] Fifth Degree

[F] Sixth degree

[G] Seventh Degree

[H] Eighth degree

[J] Nineth degree

[K] Tenth degree

Which one of the following answers above fits the description with to nerve injuries outlined as follows.

Q 3.46 A mixed nerve injury secondary to a crush injury?

Q 3.47 A localised conduction block secondary to segmental demyelination?

Q 3.48 Nerve injury usually recovers completely within 12 weeks?

Q 3.49 The nerve is in continuity but with complete scar block resulting from injury to the nerve?

Q 3.50 Axonotmesis?

QUIZ 3
ANSWERS

3.1
Answer A
Langerhan's cells form part of the immune system and function as antigen-presenting cells (APC's). Merkel cells are mechanoreceptors and melanocytes produce melanin which protect against uv radiation.

3.2
Answer D
In immature and hypertrophic scars the amount of Type 3 collagen is greater than compared to normal skin, however, the there is still a greater proportion of Type 1 collagen.

3.3
Answer C
A deficiency of Fe^{2+} or Vit C inhibits the hydroxylation of proline and lysine in the process of collagen synthesis.

3.4
Answer C
Macrophages are essential for wound healing. They act as phagocytes against microorganisms, produce cytokines such as Il-1, TNF-α and TGF- β. They attract and coordinate the activities if fibroblasts within the wound.

3.5
Answer D
Fetal wounds in the first trimester heal by regeneration rather than scarring. Inflammation and angiogensesis are reduced. There is a greater proportion of water and hyaluronic acid compared to similarly healing adult wounds.

3.6
Answer C

Bone grafts placed in a heterotopic position (the recipient site is not normally occupied by bone) are more prone to failure.

3.7
Answer B

Degree of injury	Description of nerve damage
First degree	Impaired axonal conduction but physically intact
Second degree	Axonal injury only
Third degree	Axonal injury with division of endoneurium only
Fourth degree	Division of all intraneural structures but with preservation of the epineurium
Fifth degree	Complete division of the peripheral nerve

3.8
Answer C

3.9
Answer B
Split-thickness skin grafts have less dermal elements than full-thickness grafts. As a result there is less primary contraction and greater secondary contraction than full-thickness grafts.

3.10
Answer D
Laser energy can:
- Scatter
- Reflect
- Be absorbed
- Can be transmitted through media.

3.11
Answer A
Mechanical creep involves the acute stretching of tissues. Biological creep on the other hand occurs when tissues are chronically stretched resulting in the cellular growth and cell regeneration. Stress relaxation is the plastic deformation of tissues in response to constant stress.

3.12
Answer B
Goldenhar's syndrome occurs sporadically. It is associated with hemifacial microsomia, epibulbar dermoids, vertebral abnormalities, low hairline, low set ears and accessory auricular appendages.

3.13
Answer D
Alloderm is cadaveric human dermis processed to remove all the cellular elements leaving the collagen framework. Because the cellular elements are removed it is only minimally allergenic. It is useful as a temporary skin substitute.

3.14
Answer B
The ratio of cleft lip: L : R : bilateral is 6 : 3 : 1

3.15
Answer C
Van der Woude's syndrome is an autosomal dominant condition associated with multiple pits on the lips and an absence of the second premolar tooth on the affected side.

3.16
Answer B
The levator veli palatini originates from around the Eustachian tube and inserts into the palatine aponeurosis of the soft palate. As its name suggests, it elevates the soft palate and is very important in achieving velopharyngeal closure.

3.17
Answer A
All of the muscles of the soft palate are innervated by the pharyngeal plexus except tensor veli palatini which is innervated by CN V.

3.18
Answer C
Merkel cell carcinoma has the worst prognosis of all primary skin cancers.

3.19
Answer A

Skin Type	Reaction on exposure to sunlight
I	Always burn, never tans
II	Usually burn, tans with difficulty
III	Sometimes burn
IV	Rarely burn
V	Very rarely burn, tan easily
VI	Do not burn, tans very easily

3.20
Answer B
BCCs are classified as localised, superficial and infiltrative. Morphoeic BCCs belong to the infiltrative category. Localised BCCs include nodular, nodulocystic, micronodular and pigmented BCCs.

3.21
Answer C
The 5-year survival rate from metastatic SCC is 35%.

3.22
Answer B
In a marginal excision of a soft tissue sarcoma the plane of excision runs through the pseudocapsule of the tumour. In a wide surgical excision the plane of excision extends into the normal surrounding tissues but remains within the same compartment as the tumour.

3.23
Answer D
Hirudin is secreted by leeches. It is a thrombin inhibitor.

3.24
Answer D
Regular blunt trauma is the most common cause of surface irregularity of the external secondary to haematoma formation. This is especially common in rugby players.

3.25
Answer A
Salivary gland tumours account for about 3% of all head and neck malignancies. Eighty percent of salivary gland tumours occur in the parotid gland and 80% of parotid tumours are benign.

3.26
Answer C
Warthin's tumour is a benign lesion. Ten percent of cases are bilateral. The tumour is commonly found in the tail of the parotid gland.

3.27
Answer A
Suspected metastasis from a known primary can be confirmed by an FNA. In cases where a open biopsy is indicated this should be performed via an incision along the markings for the incision for a neck dissection should this be necessary.

3.28
Answer B
The surrounding fascia of the parotid gland is an extension of the superficial layer of the deep cervical fascia.

3.29
Answer B
The facial nerve is deep to the sternocleidomastoid muscle, anterior to the posterior belly of the digastric muscle and lateral to the styloid process as it exits the stylomastoid foramen.

3.30
Answer A
The epidermis and its appendages, the nervous system and the derivatives of the neural crest cells are all derivatives of the ectoderm.

3.31
Answer B
The thyrocervical trunk does not provide a blood supply to the breast.

3.32
Answer B
The incidence of occult breast cancer in tissues excised in breast reduction is 0.06% - 0.4%.

3.33
Answer B
Regnault classification of breast ptosis:
First degree ptosis: The nipple lies above the inframammary fold
Second degree ptosis: The nipple lies below the inframammary fold but above the most dependent portion of the breast
Third degree ptosis: The nipple and the most dependent portion of the breast lies below the inframammary fold
Pseudo-ptosis: The nipple lies at the level of the inframammary fold (IMF) but the major portion of the breast tissue lies below the IMF

3.34
Answer B
Augmentation-mastopexy is an inherently difficult procedure and ideally should be done by experienced surgeons. Although it is advisable for this procedure to be done in 2 stages, it is possible to be done in one stage. It is particularly suitable for patients with an increased degree of ptosis. Although it usually involves a vertical skin incision, inverted T incisions as well as cicumareolar incisions maybe used.

3.35
Answer A
The parameters which are considered for in determining the MESS (Mangled Extremity Severity Score) to determined the salvageability of an injured limb include;
- Degree of soft tissue and skeletal injury based on the energy level of the injury
- Neurovascular assessment
- Presence of shock
- Age of the patient

A score of 7 or more suggests that salvage of the limb is improbable.

3.36
Answer B
Heprtelorism is an increased in the interorbital distance whereas, telecanthus is an increase in the intercanthal distance. Pseudotelecanthus is an illusion of telecanthus brought about prominent epicanthal folds.

3.37
Answer D
Senile (involutional) ptosis is the most common presentation of ptosis. This is due to age-related weakening of the levator aponeurosis.

3.38
Answer A
Terrestrial sunlight contains UV radiation of wavelengths between 290 and 400nm.

3.39
Answer B
Although UVB constitutes less than 0.5% of terrestrial sunlight, it is responsible for most of the photoinjury to normal skin.

3.40
Answer C
The medial fat pad is pale in colour compared to the middle fat pad in the upper eyelid.

3.41
Answer K

3.42
Answer J

3.43
Answer B

3.44
Answer G

2345
Answer H

3.46
Answer F

3.47
Answer A

3.48
Answer A

3.49
Answer D

3.50
Answer B

QUIZ 4
MULTIPLE CHOICE QUESTIONS

For questions 4.1 to 4.40 please the ONE most appropriate answer.

Q 4.1
Which ONE of the following techniques results in greatest blood loss?

[A] Liposuction

[B] Super-wet liposuction

[C] Tumescent liposuction

[D] Wet liposuction

Q 4.2
Which of the following is the most commonly injured muscle during blepharoplasty?

[A] Superior rectus muscle

[B] Superior oblique muscle

[C] Inferior rectus muscle

[D] Inferior oblique muscle

Q 4.3
Which is the following is NOT a cause for loss of vision following blepharoplasty?

[A] Injury to the inferior oblique muscle

[B] Haemorrhage

[C] Damage to eyeball during injection of local anaesthetic

[D] Excessive vasospasm from adrenaline in the local anaesthetic

Q 4.4
Which ONE of the following statements regarding vascular malformations is TRUE?

[A] They are never present at birth

[B] They usually arise a few weeks after birth

[C] They are best regarded as benign vascular tumours

[D] They never involute spontaneously

Q 4.5
Which ONE of the following can potentially penetrate deepest into the skin?

[A] UVA

[B] UVB

[C] UVC

[D] Infra-red light

Q 4.6
What is the incidence of epispadias?

[A] 1:30 live births

[B] 1:300 live births

[C] 1:3000 live births

[D] 1:30000 live births

Q 4.7
Which of the following artery runs through the lateral compartment of the leg?

[A] Anterior tibial artery

[B] Posterior tibial artery

[C] Superficial peroneal artery

[D] None of the above

Q 4.8
Which of the following statements related to compartment syndrome is TRUE?

[A] Compartment syndrome can be only diagnosed if there is an absence of a palpable distal pulse

[B] The intracompartmental pressure is greater than 30mmHg

[C] The intracompartmental pressure is more than 30mmhg below the diastolic pressure

[D] Cannot occur in traumatic injuries if the wound extends into the affected compartment

Q 4.9
Which of the following is a contraindication for free TRAM flap breast reconstruction?

[A] Pfannenstiel scar

[B] An ipsilateral paramedian scar

[C] A scar along the ipsilateral subcostal margin

[D] An appendicectomy scar following a grid-iron incision

Q 4.10
Which of the following conditions is NOT associated with gynaecomastia?

[A] Generalized obesity

[B] Hyperthyroidism

[C] Hypothyroidism

[D] Marfan's syndrome

Q 4.11
What is the nerve supply to the levator veli palatini muscle of the soft palate?

[A] CN V

[B] CN VII

[C] CN IX

[D] CN X

Q 4.12
In facial development, which of the following components is NOT a branchial arch derivative?

[A] The frontonasal process

[B] The maxillary processes

[C] The tensor veli palatini muscle

[D] The mandibular processes

Q 4.13
Which of the following structures denotes the upper border of a level III neck dissection?

[A] The posterior belly of digastric muscle

[B] The omohyoid muscle

[C] Base of the skull

[D] The bifurcation of the carotid artery

Q 4.14
With regards to mandibular reconstruction, osseointegration is NOT possible with which one of the following flaps?

[A] Free fibular osteocutaneous flap

[B] Free iliac crest osteocutaneous flap

[C] Free radial forearm osteocutaneous flap

[D] Free scapular osteocutaneous flap

Q 4.15
Which nerve listed below innervated the anterior belly of the digastrics muscle?

[A] Trigeminal nerve

[B] Facial nerve

[C] Hypoglossal nerve

[D] Lingual nerve

Q 4.16
A 73 year-old gentleman attends the outpatient's department with an enlarged level II cervical node. After further investigations, it was concluded that it was metastatic squamous cell carcinoma. Which one of the following is an unlikely site for the primary tumour?

[A] Parotid gland

[B] Floor of the mouth

[C] Oropharynx

[D] Hypopharynx

Q 4.17
The technique of recreating and/or adding definition to the antihelical fold of the pinna using nonabsorbable sutures via a postauricular incision is known as?

[A] The Mustarde technique

[B] The Furnas Technique

[C] The Gibson Technique

[D] The Stenstrom Technique

Q 4.18
What is the concentration of heparin in heparinised saline used in microsurgery?

[A] 1 unit/ml of heparin in Hartmann's solution

[B] 10 units/ml of heparin in Hartmann's solution

[C] 100 units/ml of heparin in Hartmann's solution

[D] 1000 units/ml of heparin in Hartmann's solution

Q 4.19
Which of the following is NOT a prognostic factor for soft tissue sarcomas?

[A] Size of the lesion

[B] Site of the lesion

[C] Degree of differentiation of the tumour

[D] Age of the patient

Q 4.20
Squamous cell carcinoma arise from which of the following?

[A] Cells of the basal layer of the epidermis

[B] Cells of the stratum spinosum of the epidermis

[C] Pluripotential cells of the basal layer

[D] None of the above

Q 4.21
Which of the following is NOT a premalignant lesion?

[A] Leukoplakia

[B] Actinic keratosis

[C] Bowen's disease

[D] Chronic ulcers

Q 4.22
What is the average reported rate of incomplete excision margins in the surgical treatment of BCC's?

[A] 2%

[B] 7%

[C] 12%

[D] 20%

Q 4.23
The sounds of which of the following consonants are regarded as fricatives?

[A] S

[B] B

[C] P

[D] M

Q 4.24
When performing a Furlow repair of the soft palate the base of the mucomuscular flaps are positioned?

[A] Anteriorly

[B] Posteriorly

[C] Medially

[D] Laterally

Q 4.25
Which of the following is NOT a feature of a submucous cleft?

[A] Bifid uvula

[B] Diastasis of the muscles of the soft palate in the midline with an intact oral mucosal layer

[C] Notching of the posterior hard palate

[D] Cardiovascular abnormalities

Q 4.26
Cleft lip and palate deformities are surgically primarily repaired in the first year of life. This is done for the following reasons EXCEPT?

[A] For cosmesis

[B] To improve feeding and nutrition

[C] To prevent subsequent impairment in mid-facial growth and development

[D] To prevent abnormal speech

Q 4.27
Zyderm is made up MOSTLY of which of the following type of collagen?

[A] Type 1

[B] Type 2

[C] Type 3

[D] Type 4

Q 4.28
In relation to the axis of lie of synostosed cranial sutures, cranial growth occurs?

[A] Parallel to the suture

[B] Perpendicular to the suture

[C] In multiple directions

[D] None of the above

Q 4.29
A 6 old boy who has right hemifacial microsomia presents with a severely hypoplastic right mandible. CT scan confirms the presence of a non-articulating temporo-mandibular joint. Which group of the Prozansky classification of mandibular deformity does this fall under?

[A] Group 1

[B] Group 2a

[C] Group 2b

[D] Group 3

Q 4.30
Which of the following is NOT a contraindication for the insertion of a tissue expander?

[A] Wound infection

[B] Under a skin grafted area

[C] Under a previously irradiated tissue

[D] Adjacent to a mature scar

Q 4.31
Which of the following is NOT an advantage of a split-thickness skin graft?

[A] Its surface area maybe be increased by meshing

[B] Meshing can result in less chance of haematoma or seroma formation

[C] Secondary contraction is less

[D] Conforms better to wounds with undulating surfaces

Q 4.32
Which of the following factors would adversely affect the outcome following a peripheral nerve repair with cable nerve grafts?

[A] Trimming the ends of the nerves to healthy tissue prior to repair

[B] Reversing the grafts prior to anastomosis

[C] Placing the grafts in a scarred and poorly vascularised bed

[D] Minimising the tension of the anastomoses

Q 4.33

Which one of the following is NOT performed in using the Belfast regiment of early active mobilisation following flexor tendon repair?

[A] Passive extension of the interphalangeal joints

[B] Passive flexion of the interphalangeal joints

[C] Passive flexion and hold

[D] Active flexion of the interphalangeal joints

Q 4.34

Which of the following most accurately outlines the zones of a free TRAM flap supplied by the right deep inferior epigastric artery?

From right to left

[A] 2..1..3..4

[B] 4..1..2..3

[C] 3..1..2..4

[D] 1..2..3..4

Q 4.35

Which one of the following types of cells is NOT present in the epidermis in normal healthy skin?

[A] Langerhan's cells

[B] Fibroblasts

[C] Merkel cells

[D] Melanocytes

Q 4.36
Tissue expanded skin has which one of the following properties?

[A] Utilises the elastic properties of the skin and therefore there are no new cells in the expanded tissue

[B] All of the expanded skin is composed of new cells

[C] Has an improved blood supply compared to surrounding normal skin

[D] Is asensate

Q 4.37
What is the MOST appropriate technique for the reconstruction of the entire eyebrow in a patient who underwent radiotherapy of that area?

[A] Micrograft hair follicle transplantation

[B] Hair strip grafts

[C] Pedicled postauricular temporoparietal scalp flap

[D] Scalp rotation flap

Q 4.38
Which ONE of the following techniques is NOT useful in periorbital rejuvenation?

[A] Blepharoplasty

[B] Radiotherapy

[C] Botulinum toxin

[D] Chemical peels

Q 4.39
What is the main functional muscle of the soft palate producing velopharyngeal closure?

[A] Tensor veli palatini

[B] Levator veli palatini

[C] Muscularis uvulae

[D] Stylopharyngeus

Q 4.40
What is the normal chondromastoid angle in an average adult?

[A] 5°

[B] 106°

[C] 31°

[D] 47°

QUIZ 4
EXTENDED MATCHING QUESTIONS

For questions 4.41 to 4.45 please select the ONE MOST appropriate answer from list [A] to [K]. Each answer maybe used more than once or not at all.

The following is a list of growth factors and cytokines

[A] Vascular endothelial growth factor (VEGF)
[B] Granulocyte colony-stimulating factor (G-CSF)
[C] Platelet-derived growth factor (PDGF)
[D] Keratinocyte growth factor (KGF)
[E] Epidermal growth factor (EGF)
[F] Transforming growth factor-β (TGF-β)
[G] Tumour necrosis factor-α (TNF-α)
[H] Interferon-α
[J] Interleukin-1
[K] All of the above

Q 4.41 Which of the above biologically active molecules are involved in wound healing?

Q4 4.42 Which of the above inhibits fibroblast proliferation?

Q 4.43 Which of the above induces granulopoiesis?

Q 4.44 Which of the above stimulates collagenase secretion by fibroblasts? E

Q 4.45 Which of the above induces extracellular matrix synthesis by inhibiting protease activity and up-regulating collagen and proteoglycan synthesis? F

For questions 4.46 to 4.50 please select the ONE MOST appropriate answer from list [A] to [K]. Each answer maybe used more than once or not at all.

The following is a list of facial muscles

[A] Mentalis
[B] Procerus
[C] Posterior belly of digastric
[D] Levator labii superioris alaeque nasi
[E] Levator labii superioris
[F] Zygomaticus minor
[G] Zygomaticus major
[H] Frontalis
[J] Depressor labii inferioris
[K] Masseter

Which one of the answers best fits the descriptions below

Q 4.46
All of the above facial muscles receive their innervation via their deep surfaces EXCEPT?

Q 4.47
Which one of the above muscles contributes to the glabella lines on frowning?

Q 4.48
Which one of the muscles listed above is a muscle of mastication?

Q 4.49
Which one of the muscles listed above is not muscle of facial expression although it is innervated by the facial nerve?

Q 4.50
Which one of the muscles listed above is NOT innervated by the facial nerve?

QUIZ 4
ANSWERS

4.1
Answer A
Liposction without injection of an infusant solution containing adrenaline has a blood loss of 20-45%.

4.2
Answer D
The inferior oblique muscle is the most commonly injured muascle during blepharoplasty operations.

4.3
Answer A
Injury to the inferior oblique or any extraocular muscles during blepharoplasty is more likely to result in diplopia rather than loss of vision.

4.4
Answer D
Vascular malformations are always present at birth and never involute spontaneously. Haemangiomas often arise after birth.

4.5
Answer C
The depth of penetration of light into the skin depends on the wavelength. The shorter the wavelength, the deep it penetrates. UVC has the shortest wavelength (200-290nm)of the options provided.

4.6
Answer D
The incidence of epispadias is 1:30000 live births.

4.7
Answer D
There is no major artery running through the lateral compartment of the leg.

4.8
Answer B
Compartment decompression is indicated if the intracompartmental pressure is >30mmHg or is <30mmHg below the diastolic pressure. In traumatic injuries, there is still of risk of compartment syndrome developing in the affected limb if the fascia is only partially breached (and the compartment is incompletely released). This can provide a false sense of security.

4.9
Answer C
An ipsilateral paramedian scar may indicate injury to the rectus muscle as well as the deep inferior epigastric artery.

4.10
Answer D
Gynaecomastia is associated with obesity, malnutrition, cirrhosis, renal failure, hypothyroidism and hyperthyroidism. It is not associated with Marfan's syndrome. Marfan's syndrome maybe associated with chest wall deformities.

4.11
Answer D
The levator veli palatini muscle is innervated by the vagus nerve (CN X).

4.12
Answer A
The face is formed from fusion of five processes; the frontonasal process, the paired maxillary processes and the paired mandibular processes. The maxillary and mandibular processes are derivatives of the first branchial arch. The tensor veli palatini is derived from the second branchial arch. The frontonasal process is not a branchial arch derivative.

4.13
Answer D
The superior border of level III is the bifurcation of the carotid artery, the inferior border is the omohyoid muscle, the anterior border is the posterior edge of the sternohyoid muscle and the posterior border is the posterior edge of the sternocleidomastoid muscle.

4.14
Answer C
Osteointegration is not possible with the use of the radial forearm osteocutaneous flap for mandibular reconstruction.

4.15
Answer A
The anterior belly of the digastrics muscle is innervated by the trigeminal nerve. The posterior belly in innervated by the facial nerve.

4.16
Answer B
Cancers of the floor of the mouth are likely to metastasise to level I nodes. Cancers of the oral cavity, nasal cavity, nasopharynx , oropharynx, hypopharynx, larynx and parotid gland are likely to metastasise to level II nodes.

4.17
Answer A
This is known as the Mustarde technique of prominent ear correction. The Furnas technique involves the use of concho-mastoid sutures. Stenstrom described the technique of anterior scoring to recreate the antihelical fold using the Gibson's principle (which states that if the cartilage is weakened on one side after scoring it bends away from that side).

4.18
Answer C
Heparinised saline has 100 units of heparin per ml of Hartmann's solution

4.19
Answer B
The following are the prognostic factors for soft tissue sarcomas:
- Advanced age of the patient
- Presence of metastases at the time of presentation
- Size of the lesion
- Grade and depth of the lesion

The histological grade is the most important prognostic factor.

4.20
Answer B
Squamous cell carcinoma arise from the stratum spinosum of the epidermis.

4.21
Answer D
Chronic ulcers are generally not malignant lesions although a malignancy may develop in a chronic wound after several years (average 32 years).

4.22

Answer B
The rate of incomplete excision of BCC's with surgery has been reported to be 4.7 – 7%.

4.23
Answer A
The consonants F and S are fricatives whereas B and P are plosives. M and N are nasal consonants.

4.24
Answer B
In carrying out a soft palate repair using the Furlow technique of double opposing Z-plasties, the intervening muscle layer is included in the posteriorly-based flap of each Z-plasty flap.

4.25
Answer D
The features of a submucous cleft are:
- Bifid uvula

Zona pellucidum (diastasis of the muscles of the soft palate in the midline with an intact oral mucosal layer)
- Notching of the posterior hard palate

4.26
Answer C
Cleft lip and palate procedures are undertaken for the following reasons:
- To look good
- To feed well
- For good speech
- To hear well (insertion of grommets in selected cases)
- For good dentition
- So that the patient can integrate well socially

4.27
Answer A
Zyderm is made up of collagen types 1:3 in the ration of 19:1.

4.28
Answer A
Skull growth occurs parallel to a synostosed suture eg. Synostosis of the sagittal suture results in scaphocephaly.

4.29
Answer C
The Prozansky classification of mandibular deformity is as follows:
- Group 1: Mild mandibular hypoplasia
- Group 2a: Severe mandibular hypoplasia
- Group 2b: Severe mandibular hypoplasia with a non-articulating TMJ
- Group 3: Severe mandibular hypoplasia with an absent TMJ

4.30
Answer D
The insertion of tissue expanders should be avoided in irradiated tissues, under skin grafted areas and infected areas.

4.31
Answer C

4.32
Answer C
Placing the nerve grafts in a scarred and poorly vascularised bed adversely affects the outcome. The cables should be separated from each other as they cross the defect.

4.33
Answer A
Passive extension of the interphalangeal joints in the early postoperartive period can prove to be risky and is therefore not advised.

4.34
Answer A
Zone 4 is least well perfused and is usually excised prior to the inset of the flap.

4.35
Answer B
The epidermis contains keratinocytes, Langerhan's cells, Merkel cells and melanocytes. Fibroblasts produce collagen, elastin and glycosaminoglycans (GAG's) which are all components of the dermis.

4.36
Answer C
Seventy percent of the expanded skin is due to stretch and 30% to new cells and growth. Expanded skin has an improved blood supply compared to the normal surrounding skin.

4.37
Answer C
In a poorly vascularised recipient bed, it would unsuitable to use micrograft hair transplantation or hair strip grafts. The most appropriate option would be a pedicled postauricular temporoparietal scalp flap based on the superficial temporal artery.

4.38
Answer C
In a poorly vascularised recipient bed, it would unsuitable to use micrograft hair transplantation or hair strip grafts. The most appropriate option would be a pedicled postauricular temporoparietal scalp flap based on the superficial temporal artery.

4.39
Answer B
The levator veli palatini originates from around the Eustachian tube and inserts into the palatine aponeurosis of the soft palate. As its name suggests, it elevates the soft palate and is very important in achieving velopharyngeal closure.

4.40
Answer C
The normal chondromastoid angle in an average adult is about 31.1° based on work by Da Silva Freitas et al.

2.41
Answer K

2.42
Answer H

2.43
Answer B

2.44
Answer E

2.45
Answer F

2.46
Answer F

2.47
Answer B

2.48
Answer K

2.49
Answer C

2.50
Answer K

QUIZ 5
MULTIPLE CHOICE QUESTIONS

For questions 5.1 to 5.40 please the ONE most appropriate answer.

Q 5.1
With regards to free tissue transfer, which of the following statements is true?

[A] It is absolutely contraindicated in elderly patients

[B] Preoperative radiation is a contraindication

[C] Patients must be heparinized

[D] Is possible using previously irradiated vessels

Q 5.2
At what age would you consider performing a total ear reconstruction for a newborn with severe unilateral microtia?

[A] In the first weeks of life

[B] At 1 year of age

[C] At 6 years of age

[D] At 12 years of age

Q 5.3
Following a left neck dissection for nodal metastases of a 4.3mm Breslow thickness melanoma of the left cheek, the patient develops a 'milky' ooze from the wound. What is the appropriate management of this?

[A] Leave alone, it should settle spontaneously

[B] Prompt surgical re-exploration and attempt to repair the damaged lymphatic duct

[C] Regular change of dressing with the administration of intravenous antibiotics

[D] Place the patient on a fat-free diet initially

Q 5.4
A 65 year old patient had a poorly differentiated excised from the right chhek 1 year ago, now presents with an enlarged solitary lymph node. What is the next step in the management of this patient?

[A] A CT scan of the neck and chest

[B] An FNA of the enlarged lymph node and arranging a CT scan of the neck and chest

[C] An open biopsy of the enlarged lymph node

[D] Proceed to a modified radical neck dissection

Q 5.5
Which ONE of the following nerves is not anatomically related to the submandibular gland?

[A] Marginal mandibular nerve

[B] Hypoglossal nerve

[C] Spinal accessory nerve

[D] Lingual nerve

Q 5.6
A 65 year-old gentleman presents with a right sided lagophthalmos, hyperacusis, a droopy right cheek and drooling from the right corner of the mouth. He is able to wrinkle his forehead on upward gaze. It has been determined that he has a lesion of the facial nerve. At what level is the lesion?

[A] Cortical

[B] The nucleus of the facial nerve

[C] Intratemporal

[D] At the stylomastoid foramen

Q 5.7
Which of the following signs is indicative of a parotid tumour infiltrating into the facial nerve?

[A] Hyperacusis

[B] Altered sensation over the forehead on the ipsilateral side

[C] Drooling from the corner of the mouth on the ipsilateral side

[D] Loss of taste to the anterior two-thirds of the tongue

Q 5.8
Branches of the facial nerve innervate the muscles of facial expression. It enters the following muscles on their superficial surface except?

[A] Mentalis

[B] Buccinator

[C] Levator anguli superioris

[D] Depressor anguli oris

Q 5.9
The external auditory canal is a derivative of the following embryological structures?

[A] The first branchial arch

[B] The fist branchial cleft

[C] The second branchial arch

[D] The second branchial cleft

Q 5.10
Which of the following conditions is NOT associated with an increased risk of breast cancer?

[A] Peutz-Jeghers syndrome

[B] Poland's syndrome

[C] Mutation of the BRCA2 gene

[D] Cowden disease

Q 5.11
With regards to breast reconstruction which of the following statements is FALSE?

[A] The risk of recurrence of breast cancer for women who have undergone breast reconstruction and those who have not is the same

[B] Breast reconstruction does not impede the ability of detection of a recurrence

[C] Immediate breast reconstruct is contraindicated in women who are certain to receive adjuvant radiotherapy

[D] The aesthetic outcome of immediate breast reconstruction is usually better than a delayed reconstruction

Q 5.12
Which of the following statements MOST accurately describes a subcutaneous mastectomy?

[A] Excision of all of the breast tissue and the overlying skin

[B] Excision of the breast tissue preserving the overlying skin

[C] Excision of most of the breast tissue preserving the nipple-areolar complex and overlying skin

[D] Excision of the breast and nipple-areolar complex and preserving the overlying skin flaps

Q 5.13
Which of the following is an accurate description of a Grade IIIc lower limb injury based on the Gustilo and Anderson classification?

[A] A high energy injury with extensive soft tissue damage

[B] A high energy injury with extensive soft tissue damage with periosteal stripping and bone exposure

[C] A high energy injury with extensive soft tissue damage, bony exposure and division of the tibial vessels

[D] A high energy injury with extensive soft tissue damage, bony exposure requiring soft tissue coverage with injury to the tibial nerve

Q 5.14
A 20 year patient presents with an open fracture of the left tibia with a 10cm gaping wound on the anterior aspect of the left leg. He is taken to theatre within 6 hours and the wound is adequately debrided left open and also undergoes internal fixation of the fractured tibia. Five hours post-operatively he complains of severe pain in the limb. A diagnosis of compartment syndrome is arrived at and he taken to theatre for fasciotomy. How many compartments need to be decompressed in this patient?

[A] 2

[B] 3

[C] 4

[D] 5

Q 5.15
Botulinum toxin is useful in treatment of all of the following except?

[A] Static wrinkles of the cheek

[B] Glabella lines

[C] Hyperdrosis of the axillae

[D] Anal fissures

Q 5.16
Which of the following statements is true regarding the relationship between smoking and free TRAM flaps?
[A] There is an increased rate of thrombosis at the anastomotic site in smokers

[B] There is an increased rate of flap loss in smokers

[C] There is an increased rate of fat necrosis in smokers

[D] There is an increased rate of partial flap necrosis and wound breakdown in smokers

Q 5.17
Which of the following statements concerning hypospadias is TRUE?

[A] About 50% of cases are associated with inguinal hernias

[B] About 50% of cases are associated with undescended testes

[C] Undescended testes may indicate an intersex state

[D] Most cases of hypospadias are proximal

Q 5.18
A 9-month old infant is seen in the outpatient's clinic with a 2.5cm in diameter fleshy-looking non-ulcerated vascular lesion which appear 3 weeks after birth and has been steadily increasing in size since. It is now encroaching onto the lateral aspect of the upper eyelid but does not appear to cause ptosis. What would be the most appropriate mode of treatment for this patient?

[A] Urgent surgical intervention

[B] Urgent ophalmological review and commencement of a course of systemic steroids after laising with a paediatrician

[C] Refer the infant to an interventional radiologist for urgent selective embolization

[D] Do nothing and wait for the haemangioma to resolve spontaneously

Q 5.19
You are called to the neonatal unit to see a 5-hour old infant with a hugh bluish lesion occupying most of the anterior and lateral aspects of the right thigh. You are told than the neonate is severely thrombopenic with an abnormal clotting screen, reduced fibrinogen levels and elevated levels of fibrin degradation products. What is the most likely diagnosis?

[A] Severe sickle cell anaemia

[B] Haemangioendothelioma

[C] Large arteriovenous malformation

[D] Idiopathic thrombocytopenia

Q 5.20
Which ONE of the following ranges of wavelengths best describes the wavelength of visible light?

[A] 290-400nm

[B] 400–700nm

[C] 700-850nm

[D] More than 900nm

Q 5.21
Which ONE of the following is not a constituent of sunscreens?

[A] PABA and its esters

[B] Salicylates

[C] Benzophenones

[D] Psoralens

Q 5.22
How many fat compartments are there in the lower eyelid?

[A] 1

[B] 2

[C] 3

[D] 4

Q 5.23
Which ONE of the following is NOT a function of the inferior oblique muscle?

[A] External rotation

[B] Elevation

[C] Oblique rotation

[D] Abduction

Q 5.24
Which of the following is the MOST common structure to be damaged during facelift surgery?

[A] The frontal branch of the facial nerve

[B] The zygomatic branch of the facial nerve

[C] The marginal mandibular branch of the facial nerve

[D] The great auricular nerve

Q 5.25
Liposuction carried out with an infusion of a solution of normal saline, lidocaine and adrenaline. What is the name given to the technique when the infusant to aspirate ratio is 1:1?

[A] Liposuction

[B] Wet liposuction

[C] Super-wet liposuction

[D] Tumescent liposuction

Q 5.26
The Trojani classification of soft tissue sarcomas involves all of the following parameters EXCEPT?

[A] Size of the lesion

[B] Degree of necrosis

[C] Degree of differentiation

[D] Mitotic index

Q 5.27
Which of the following is NOT a contraindication for sentinel lymph node biopsy in a patient with malignant melanoma of the lower leg?

[A] A patient who has already had a wider a wider excision and the defect reconstructed

[B] There is no clinical evidence of inguinal lymphadenopathy

[C] Pregnancy

[D] Evidence of systemic metastases

Q 5.28
A 10 year-old patient presents with a large blue-grey pigmented patch on the right shoulder area which has been present from birth. What is this MOST likely to be?

[A] Naevus of Ito

[B] Naevus of Oto

[C] Large blue naevus

[D] Mongolian spot

Q 5.29
A 43 year female patient presents with a darkly pigmented ulcerated lesion on her left thigh. An excisional biopsy was performed and the histological report stated that the lesion was a malignant melanoma of Breslow thickness 3.5mm. She had no enlarged inguinal lymphadenopathy. According to the AJCC staging system for malignant melanoma which of the following is the appropriate stage of the case outlined above assuming that she had no distant metastases?

[A] Stage IB

[B] Stage IIB

[C] Stage IIIA

[D] Stage IIIB

Q 5.30
What the MOST likely overall 5-year survival for the above patient?

[A] 30%

[B] 50%

[C] 60%

[D] 80%

Q 5.31
The histological classification used to group SCC's based on their degree of differentiation is known by which of the following?

[A] Breslow's classification

[B] Broder's classification

[C] Clark's classification

[D] Trojani classification

Q 5.32
Which of the following is a disadvantage of using the Millard rotation advancement technique in repairing a cleft lip?

[A] The vertical scar is concealed by the philtral column

[B] The horizontal scar is placed across the nasal sill

[C] There is room to adjust the height of the lip during surgery

[D] The repair can be revised with relative ease by re-elevation and re-rotation of the flaps

Q 5.33
With regards to the treatment of bilateral cleft lip which of the following statements is CORRECT?

[A] Presurgical orthopaedic appliances are always used

[B] The prolabium is the skeletal remnant of the medial nasal processes of the frontonasal process

[C] The Millard technique of cleft lip repair cannot be used since it is useful in unilateral cleft lip repair

[D] The Manchester repair is used when the prolabium is relatively small

Q 5.34
What is the blood supply to the hard palate?

[A] Lesser palatine artery

[B] Greater palatine artery

[C] Ascending pharyngeal artery

[D] Ascending palatine branch of the facial artery

Q 5.35
What is Zyplast?

[A] Is a synthetic polymer

[B] An injectable filler composed of short polymer chains of silicone

[C] An injectable filler composed of polymer chains of silicone with a high degree of cross-linking with glycosaminoglycan chains

[D] An injectable filler composed of collagen cross-linked with glutaraldehyde

Q 5.36
All of the following are clinical features of true plagiocephaly EXCEPT?

[A] The skull is triangular shaped

[B] Prominence of the ipsilateral cheek

[C] The distance between the lateral orbit and the ear is decreased on the ipsilateral side

[D] Prominence of the contralateral brow

Q 5.37
Which of the following is NOT a feature of Albright's syndrome?

[A] Precocious puberty

[B] Polyostotic fibrous dysplasia

[C] Pituitary tumours

[D] Multiple neurofibromas

Q 5.38
Which of the following is NOT a disadvantage of using tissue expanders?

[A] Involves at least 2 operations and multiple outpatient clinic appointments

[B] The expanded skin is asensate

[C] Temporary cosmetic deformity

[D] Risks of infection and expander extrusion

Q 5.39
A new Class IV Nd:YAG laser is available for use in your department. Which of the following statements is TRUE?

[A] Lasers are rated by their potential to induce ocular damage

[B] Lasers are rated by their depth of penetrance of solid lead shields

[C] The smoke fumes generated by the use of lasers are not as hazardous as that produced by electrocautery

[D] Flammable liquids can be safely used with lasers since the heat produced is deep within the tissues

Q 5.40
A free vascularised fibula used to reconstruct a tibial defect mainly heals by which one of the following processes?

[A] Osseoconduction

[B] Incorporation

[C] Oseoinduction

[D] Osteogenesis

QUIZ 5
EXTENDED MATCHING QUESTIONS

For questions 5.41 to 5.45 please select the ONE MOST appropriate answer from list [A] to [K]. Each answer maybe used more than once or not at all.

The following is a list of conditions which may affect the skin.

[A] Xeroderma pigmentosum
[B] Dystrophic epidermolysis bullosa
[C] Cutis laxa
[D] Pseudoxanthoma elasticum
[E] Ehlos-Danlos syndrome
[F] Acne vulgaris
[G] Acne rosacea
[H] Hydradenitis suppurativa
[J] Pyoderma gangrenosum
[K] Rhinophyma

Which one of the following answers above fits best for the questions outlined below.

Q5.41
Chronic infection of the apocrine sweat glands?

Q 5.42
Is associated with abnormal wound healing?

Q 5.43
Associated with superficial abscesses and ulceration secondary to a necrotising vasculitis?

Q 5.44
An autosomal recessive disorder?

Q 5.45
Affected patients have more than 1000 times more skin cancers than the normal population?

For questions 5.46 to 5.50 please select the ONE MOST appropriate answer from list [A] to [K]. Each answer maybe used more than once or not at all.

The following is a list of the various types of open fractures based on the Gustilo classification.

[A] Type I
[B] Type II
[C] Type III
[D] Type IIIA
[E] Type IIIB
[F] Type IIIC
[G] Type IIID
[H] Type IV
[J] Closed fracture
[K] None of the above

Please the descriptions below to the appropriate type of fracture.

Q 5.46
An open fracture of the humerus associated with a wound of 2cm with injury to the posterior tibial artery but no extensive soft tissue damage?

Q 5.47
An open fracture of the tibia associated with soft tissue loss, periosteal stripping and bone exposure?

Q 5.48
An open fracture of the tibia with a wound of 3cm without extensive soft-tissue damage?

Q 5.49
An open fracture of the tibia with injury to the anterior tibial artery?

Q 5.50
An open fracture of the tibia with a 2cm wound without extensive soft tissue damage with injury to the common peroneal nerve but with intact vessels?

QUIZ 5
ANSWERS

5.1
Answer D
It is possible to perform free tissue transfer using recipient vessels which have been previously taken, however great care needs to be exercised.

5.2
Answer C
The rib cartilages used in total ear reconstruction are only large enough in children 6 years of age to create an adult size ear.

5.3
Answer D
This represents a chyle leak secondary to an injury to the thoracic duct and should be treated conservatively with a fat-free diet initially. If it fails to subside TPN may prove useful.

5.4
Answer A
The disease needs to be staged by obtaining a histological/cytological diagnosis and a staging CT scan to rule out distant metastases. If the FNA results reveal evidence of metastases and there is no distant metastases detected by the staging scan, then the patient should undergo a neck dissection.

5.5
Answer C
The spinal accessory nerve is not closely related to the submandibular gland.

5.6
Answer C
In this case the function of the frontalis muscle is intact on the affected side. Hence, this is a lower motor neurone lesion distal to the nucleus of the facial nerve. The nerve to the stapedius muscle is involved (hence the hyperacusis). This is an intratemporal branch of the facial nerve. Hence, this lesion is most certainly intratemporal.

5.7
Answer C
The facial nerve branches within the substance of the parotid gland into five branches to innervate the muscles of facial expression.

5.8
Answer D
The facial nerve usually enter the muscles of facial expression on their deep surface except the mentalis, buccinator and the levator anguli superioris where it enters on the superficial surface.

5.9
Answer B
The external auditory canal is a derivative of the first branchial cleft.

5.10
Answer B
The following conditions predispose to an increased risk of breast cancer.
- Mutations of the BRCA 1 and 2 genes
- Peutz-Jeghers syndrome
- Cowden disease
- Li-Fraumeni syndrome

5.11
Answer C
Immediate breast reconstruct is not contraindicated in women who are certain to receive adjuvant radiotherapy. The risk of recurrence of breast cancer for women who have undergone breast reconstruction and those who have not is the same and breast reconstruction does not impede the ability of detection of a recurrence. The aesthetic outcome of immediate breast reconstruction is usually better than a delayed reconstruction because the natural breast contour is better preserved.

5.12
Answer C
Subcutaneous mastectomy involves excision of most of the breast tissue preserving the nipple-areolar complex and overlying skin. Skin-sparing mastectomy, on the other hand, involves excision of the breast and nipple-areolar complex and preserving the overlying skin flaps.

5.13
Answer C
A Grade IIIc lower limb limb injury, according to the Gustilo and Anderson classification, involves an open lower limb fracture with arterial injury requiring repair.

5.14
Answer C
The fascial compartments of the leg are the anterior, peroneal and superficial and deep posterior compartments. Despite the presence of the anterior wound, all four compartments need to be formally decompressed.

5.15
Answer A
Botox is not useful for the treatment of static wrinkles in areas such as the cheek. Although botulinum toxin is useful in the treatment of anal fissures it is not specifically licensed for this use.

5.16
Answer D
There is an increased rate of partial flap necrosis and wound breakdown in smokers. There is no increase in the rates of anastomotic thrombosis, flap loss or flap necrosis in smokers.

5.17
Answer C
Hypospadias with undescended testes may indicate an intersex state. About 9% of cases of hypospadias present with inguinal hernias and a similar proportion of cases with undescended testes. These increase with more proximal hypospadias.

5.18
Answer B
In this case the lesion has not started to spontaneously resolve and is still in its growth phase. Doing nothing and waiting expectantly for it to resolve is not an option since it can potentially still enlarge to obstruct vision which can result in amblyopia and anisometropia. An urgent ophalmological review and commencement of a course of systemic steroids after laising with a paediatrician is indicated here.

5.19
Answer B
This is a classical description of the Kasabach-Merritt syndrome due to a haemangioendothelioma. The description given is of thrombocytopenia with disseminated intravascular coagulation (DIC).

5.20
Answer B
The wavelength of visible light is between 400 – 700nm.

5.21
Answer D
The constituents of sunscreens include PABA and its esters, salicylates, cinnamates, anthranilates, benzophenones, dibenzoylmethanes and benzylidene camphors. Psoralens are a photosensitising agent found in plants. It is a light-sensitive compound, when exposed to UVA light, can become toxic to certain malignant or disease cells.

5.22
Answer C
There are 3 fat compartments in the lower eyelid.

5.23
Answer C
The primary action of the inferior oblique muscle is external rotation of the eyeball. The secondary action is elevation and the tertiary action is abduction.

5.24
Answer D
Although the branches of the facial nerves maybe injured during facelift operations and the results maybe dire (particularly if the frontal or marginal mandibular branches are involved), the most commonly injured nerve during this procedure is the great auricular nerve.

5.25
Answer C
Super-wet liposuction uses the same fluid injection as the tumescent technique but has an infusant to aspirate ratio of 1:1. The tumescent technique has a ratio of 2:1 or 3:1.

5.26
Answer A
This classification is based on histological analysis.

5.27
Answer B
The following are contraindications for SLNB:
- Lymphadenopathy in the related draining basin
- Patients with evidence of systemic metastasis
- Patients with melanoma less than pT1b
- Patients who have already undergone a wider local excision
- The radioactive dye should not be used during pregnancy although the blue dye is not contraindicated
- Allergy to the blue dye
- SLNB maybe difficult to perform in the head and neck because of the proximity of the lesion to the lymph nodes and the tendency for the lymph to be present in clusters

5.28
Answer A
This is classical of a naevus of Ito. It is more common in people of Oriental Origin. A naevus of Oto typically presents on the face in the periorbital area and may involve the conjunctiva.

5.29
Answer B
This is a T3b, N0, M0 tumour which is an AJCC Stage IIB.

5.30
Answer C

5.31
Answer B
Broder's classification is based on histological analysis and is denoted by the ratio of differentiated to undifferentiated cells.
Grade 1:   3 : 1
Grade 2:   1 : 1
Grade 3:   1 : 3
Grade 4:   Tumour has no tendency towards differentiation

5.32
Answer B
With the Millard's technique for cleft lip repair, one of the main disadvantages is the placement of the horizontal scar across the nasal sill. The advantages of the technique are:
- The vertical scar is concealed by the philtral column
- There is room to adjust the height of the lip during surgery hence, it is known as the 'cut as you go' technique
- The repair can be revised with relative ease by re-elevation and re-rotation of the flaps

5.33
Answer D
In bilateral cleft lip the prolabium is the soft tissue remnant of the medial nasal processes of the frontonasal process. The skeletal element is the premaxilla. If the prolabium is relatively large, the Millard repair can be used. If the prolabium is relatively small the Manchester repair is used.

5.34
Answer B
The greater palatine artery which is a branch of the maxillary artery is supplies the hard palate.

5.35
Answer D
Zyplast is an injectable filler composed of collagen cross-linked with glutaraldehyde. It is used to treat coarse rhytids and is longer lasting than Zyderm.

5.36
Answer B
In' true' plagiocephaly the skull is shaped like a rhomboid (or parallelogram) whereas in 'positional' plagiocephaly the skull is shaped like a triangle with its apex lying on the affected side.

5.37
Answer D
Albright's syndrome is characterised by polyostotic fibrous dysplasia (multiple bony lesions), precocious puberty, pituitary tumours and cafe-au-lait spots.

5.38
Answer B
The expanded skin usually has similar degree of sensation as the surrounding skin.

5.39
Answer A
Lasers are rated by their potential to induce ocular damage. Because the smoke fumes may contain traces of blood and potentially viruses, special laser quality masks must be worn. Flammable prep must not be used.

5.40
Answer D
This is the predominant process whereby vascularised bone grafts heal by the formation of new bone by the osteocytes within the graft itself.

5.41
Answer H

5.42
Answer E

5.43
Answer J

5.44
Answer A

133

5.45
Answer A

5.46
Answer F

5.47
Answer E

5.48
Answer B

5.49
Answer F

5.50
Answer B

QUIZ 6
MULTIPLE CHOICE QUESTIONS

For questions 6.1 to 6.40 please the ONE most appropriate answer.

Q 6.1

What is the dominant type of collagen in normal skin?

[A] Type 1 collagen

[B] Type 3 collagen

[C] Type 5 collagen

[D] Type 4 collagen

Q 6.2

When comparing the histological properties of the skin of the skin of a 90 year-old female to a 20 year old female which of the following is most likely to be true?

[A] The dermis would appear thicker due to chronic sun damage

[B] Flattening of the dermo-epidermal junction

[C] A general increased density of melonocytes resulting in a more pigmented appearance

[D] Thickening of the stratum corneum of the epidermis

Q 6.3

In which of the following patients it would be safe to perform an elective facelift procedure?

[A] A patient with cutis laxa

[B] A patient with progeria

[C] A patient with Ehlers-Danlos syndrome

[D] None of the above

Q 6.4
Which of the following statements is FALSE regarding the role of TGF-β in normal wound healing?

[A] Attracts fibroblasts into the wound

[B] Stimulates collagen production by fibroblasts

[C] Stimulates angiogenesis

[D] Is produced by macrophages and does not play a role in the attraction of macrophages into the wound

Q 6.5
Which of the following is not essential for wound healing?

[A] Vitamin A

[B] Vitamin C

[C] Vitamin D

[D] Vitamin E

Q 6.6
A 65 year old gentleman presents with a chronic wound on his left shin where he previously had radiotherapy for a basal cell carcinoma. Which of statements is FALSE?

[A] Radiotherapy results in arteritis obliterans leading to poor wound healing

[B] Radiotherapy may have damaged the lymphatics of the tissue predisposing the wound to an increased risk of infection

[C] Following radiotherapy for the BCC the current wound is not due to a recurrence of the malignancy

[D] Radiotherapy results in decreased collagen production and hence poor wound healing

Q 6.7
Skin grafts placed on well vascularised beds usually fail because of the following reasons EXCEPT?

[A] The area is denervated

[B] Haematoma under graft

[C] Infected wound

[D] Mechanical shear on the graft in the early stages

Q 6.8
With regards to the structure of cortical bone, each individual bone unit called an osteon comprises all of the following EXCEPT?

[A] Osteocytes

[B] A central nutrient blood vessel

[C] A haversian canal

[D] A Volkmann's canal

Q 6.9
Lasers use the technique of selective photothermolysis. What is the chromophore for the Nd:YAG laser when used for hair removal?

[A] Water

[B] Haemoglobin

[C] Melanin

[D] Collagen

Q 6.10
How is the diameter of an expander estimated?

[A] Should be the same as the diameter of the defect

[B] Should be 3.14 times the diameter of the defect

[C] Should be 2.5 times the diameter of the defect

[D] Should be 5 times the diameter of the defect

Q 6.11
The gain in the area of tissue obtained through expansion is influenced by the shape of the expander. Which of the following shapes of expanders produces the maximal gain in surface area of the expanded skin?

[A] Round

[B] Oval

[C] Crescentic

[D] Rectangular

Q 6.12
Which one of the following Tessier clefts is not a feature in Treacher Collins syndrome?

[A] Cleft no. 6

[B] Cleft no. 7

[C] Cleft no. 8

[D] Cleft no. 9

Q 6.13
Which of the following is characteristic of Romberg's hemifacial atrophy?

[A] It presents after 5 years of age

[B] It has an autosomal pattern of inheritance

[C] It is associated with a positive family history

[D] The underlying bony skeleton is characteristically not affected

Q 6.14
Premature fusion of the cranial sutures results in an abnormality of skull morphology. Which of the following is the MOST common skull morphology associated with synostosis?

[A] Phagiocephaly

[B] Scaphocephaly

[C] Trigonocephaly

[D] Brachycephaly

Q 6.15
All of the following are clinical features of true plagiocephaly EXCEPT?

[A] The skull is triangular shaped

[B] Prominence of the ipsilateral cheek

[C] The distance between the lateral orbit and the ear is decreased on the ipsilateral side

[D] Prominence of the contralateral brow

Q 6.16
Which of the following is a feature of allografts?

[A] Tissue derived from a different species

[B] Non-living tissue derived from a member of the same species

[C] Non-living tissue derived from a member of a different species

[D] Preserved non-living tissue derived from the same individual

Q 6.17
Which of the following is NOT a feature of isolated cleft palate?

[A] More common in females

[B] More likely to be associated with a syndrome than patients with cleft lip and palate

[C] Usually bilateral

[D] More likely to be associated with environmental causes than familial factors

Q 6.18
Which of the following is NOT a characteristic feature of a complete cleft lip deformity?

[A] Decrease in the vertical height of the upper lip

[B] There is no nasal deformity in a significant proportion of cases

[C] Abnormal insertion of the orbicularis oris into the nasal spine and alar base

[D] A cleft of the hard palate anterior to the incisive foramen

Q 6.19
What is the primary abnormality that results in the Pierre-Robin sequence?

[A] Failure of rotation of the palatal shelves

[B] Failure of the tongue to descend

[C] A small jaw

[D] Failure of fusion of the palatal shelves resulting in a U-shaped cleft palate

Q 6.20
Which of the following statements regarding giant congenital hairy naevii is TRUE?

[A] Histologically, they are confined to the epidermis

[B] They remain the same size from birth and characteristically do not grow in proportion to the body size

[C] They are not confined to the dermis and may invade into underlying muscle and bone

[D] They are benign lesions and do not carry any risk of malignant transformation

Q 6.21
Which of the following is the most common type of skin cancer?

[A] Basal cell carcinoma

[B] Squamous cell carcinoma

[C] Merkel cell carcinoma

[D] Malignant melanoma

Q 6.22
Pigmented BCC's arise from which of the following cell types?

[A] The pluripotential cells of the epithelium at the dermoepidermal junction

[B] Melanocytes with the basal layer of the epidermis

[C] Keratinocytes within the basal layer of the epidermis

[D] Keratinocytes from the granular layer of the epidermis

Q 6.23
Which of the following is NOT true of keratoacanthomas?

[A] They demonstrate rapid growth

[B] They can resolve spontaneously

[C] Can be easily differentiated from squamous cell carcinomas by histological examination

[D] They are associated with the Ferguson-Smith syndrome

Q 6.24
The histological classification used to group SCC's based on their degree of differentiation is known by which of the following?

[A] Breslow's classification

[B] Broder's classification

[C] Clark's classification

[D] Trojani classification

Q 6.25
The histology report for a patient with a malignant melanoma of the right anterior chest wall indicated that the tumour extended to junction of the papillary and reticular dermis. This corresponds to which of the following?

[A] At least a Breslow thickness of 2.0mm

[B] At least a Breslow thickness of 1.0 mm

[C] Clark's level 3

[D] Clark's level

Q 6.26
On attempting to replant the tip of the right index finger in a 30 year-old accountant, despite patent arterial and venous anastomoses no perfusion is noted in the replanted part. Which of the following statements is TRUE?

[A] This is most likely due to a technical problem

[B] The patient should be heparinized

[C] This is due to the no-reflow phenomenon

[D] This is most likely due to the combined effect of the anaesthetic drugs

Q 6.27
Which of the following most accurately outlines the mechanism of action of heparin?

[A] Inhibits platelet aggregation through the inhibition of cyclooxygenase

[B] Inactivates Von Willebrand factor

[C] Increases the number of mast cells

[D] Inhibits thrombin and factor Xa by binding to antithrombin III

Q 6.28
At what age would you consider performing a total ear reconstruction for a newborn with severe unilateral microtia?

[A] In the first weeks of life

[B] At 1 year of age

[C] At 6 years of age

[D] At 12 years of age

Q 6.29
Which of the following statements is TRUE about magnetic resonance imaging (MRI)?

[A] Its mode of action depends on high frequency sound waves

[B] In T1-weighted images water appears as white

[C] In T2-weighted images fat appear white

[D] MRI is superior to CT imaging for demonstrating areas of inflammation within tissues

Q 6.30
Which of the following statements regarding adenoid cystic carcinoma of the parotid gland is TRUE?

[A] The facial nerve is prone to invasion

[B] Is the most common malignant tumour of the parotid gland

[C] Has a low propensity for recurrence and metastases

[D] Usually presents bilaterally

Q 6.31
A 93 year-old female patient with significant coronary artery disease underwent a segmental mandibulectomy of the lateral segment (not involving the condyle) for an intraoral squamous cell carcinoma. The defect is 10cm in width. What is the MOST appropriate method to reconstruct the defect?

[A] Bridging contoured reconstruction plate and coverage with free radial forearm flap

[B] Bridging contoured reconstruction plate and coverage with local soft tissues

[C] Non-vascularised free bone graft

[D] Free fibula flap

Q 6.32
Which of the following nerves does NOT provide sensory innervation to the nose?

[A] Infraorbital nerve

[B] Infratrochlear nerve

[C] Nasociliary nerve

[D] Buccal branch of CN VII

145

Q 6.33
A 65 year-old gentleman presents with a right sided lagophthalmos, hyperacusis, a droopy right cheek and drooling from the right corner of the mouth. He is able to wrinkle his forehead on upward gaze. It has been determined that he has a lesion of the facial nerve. At what level is the lesion?

[A] Cortical

[B] The nucleus of the facial nerve

[C] Intratemporal

[D] At the stylomastoid foramen

Q 6.34
Which of the following are derivatives of the second branchial arch?

[A] The muscles of mastication

[B] The muscles of facial expression

[C] The mandible

[D] The maxilla

Q 6.35
What is the nerve supply to the stylopharyngeus muscle?

[A] The trigeminal nerve

[B] The facial nerve

[C] The glossopharyngeal nerve

[D] The hypoglossal nerve

Q 6.36
Which of the following vessels provides the dominant blood supply to the breast?

[A] Internal thoracic artery

[B] Lateral thoracic artery

[C] Lateral branches of the intercostals arteries

[D] Thoracodorsal artery

Q 6.37
A slim, athletic 38year-old woman presents requesting a delayed left breast reconstruction. She did not undergo radiotherapy following her mastectomy. She would like the size of the reconstructed breast to match her right breast which is D-cup in size. What is the MOST appropriate method of reconstruction which should be offered to this patient?

[A] A breast implant reconstruction

[B] A breast expander reconstruction followed by exchange for a definitive implant after expansion

[C] A pedicled latissimus dorsi muscle reconstruction

[D] A DIEP flap reconstruction

Q 6.38
Which of the following flaps is NOT suitable for the coverage of defects around the knee?

[A] Pedicled soleus flap

[B] Medial gastocnenius muscle flap

[C] Lateral gastrocnemius muscle flap

[D] Saphenous fasciocutaneous flap

Q 6.39
Which of the following is NOT a licensed use of botulinum toxin?

[A] Static wrinkles on the cheek

[B] Glabella lines

[C] Hyperhidrosis of the axillae

[D] Blepharospasm

Q 6.40
Which of the following is not an indication for treatment of haemangiomas?

[A] Obstruction of the visual axis for one week

[B] Increase in size of the lesion

[C] Ulceration and frequent episodes of bleeding

[D] A glottis lesion presenting with stridor

QUIZ 6
EXTENDED MATCHING QUESTIONS

For questions 6.41 to 6.45 please select the ONE MOST appropriate answer from list [A] to [K]. Each answer maybe used more than once or not at all.

[A] Epidermis

[B] Pilosebaceous unit

[C] Apocrine unit

[D] Eccrine sweat glands

[E] Langerhan's cells

[F] Melanocytes

[G] Macrophages

[H] Merkel cells

[J] Blood vessels

[K] Fibroblasts

Q 6.41
Which of the following are all embryologically derived from the ectoderm?
[a] A,B F,J
[b] A,C,B,D
[c] F,G,H,K
[d] A,B,F,H

Q 6.42
Which one of the above is embryologically derived from the neuroectoderm?

Q 6.43
Which of the following is embryologically derived from the mesoderm?
[a] C,D,E,F
[b] F,G,H,K
[c] G,H,K ,J
[d] C,D,E,J

Q 6.44
Which one of the following groups best outlines cells of the epidermis?
[a] F,K
[b] H,K
[c] E,K
[d] E,H

Q 6.45
Which one of the above cells produces collagen?

For questions 6.46 to 6.50 please select the ONE MOST appropriate answer from list [A] to [K]. Each answer maybe used more than once or not at all.

The following is a list of craniofacial conditions.

[A] Crouzon syndrome
[B] Apert syndrome
[C] Pfeiffer syndrome
[D] Saethre-Chozen syndrome
[E] Carpenter syndrome
[F] Moebius syndrome
[G] Fibrous dysplasia
[H] Romberg disease
[J] Treacher Collins syndrome
[K] Plexiform neurofibroma

Please match one of the conditions listed above with the most suitable answer for the questions below.

Q 6.46
Congenital paralysis of the sixth and seventh cranial nerves?

Q 6.47
An autosomal dominant condition associated with craniosynostosis, broad thumbs and broad great toes?

Q 6.48
An autosomal dominant condition with craniosynostosis but no abnormalities of the hands?

Q 6.49
An autosomal dominant condition with symmetric syndactyly of both hands and feet?

Q 6.50
Associated with progressive hemifacial atrophy of unknown aetiology?

QUIZ 6
ANSWERS

6.1
Answer A
Type 1 collagen is the dominant type in normal skin (Type 1 : Type 3 is 5:1). Type 2 collagen is present in hyaline cartilage. Types 4 and 5 collagen are present in the basement membrane of the epidermis.

6.2
Answer B
In the aging skin there is flattening of the dermo-epidermal junctions, dermal atrophy and a decreased density of melanocytes.

6.3
Answer A
Patients with cutis laxa present with features of premature aging due to loose, inelastic skin. They don't have wound healing problems.

6.4
Answer D
TGF-β is a growth factor which attracts both fibroblasts and macrophages. It stimulates the production of extracellar matrix by fibroblasts and induces angiogenesis.

6.5
Answer C
Deficiencies of vitamins A, C and E result in poor wound healing. Vitamin C is required for collagen synthesis and vitamin E is a membrane stabilizer. Vitamin D is important in calcium metabolism.

6.6
Answer C
Radiotherapy damages the small blood vessels of the tissue (arteritis obliterans) resulting in decreased tissue perfusion. It can also damage the lymphatics and the fibroblasts (resulting in a decreased production of collagen). The chronic wound may be due to recurrence of the BCC (since radiotherapy has a 92% cure rate) or even a marjolin's ulcer.

6.7
Answer A
Although denervation may contribute to delayed wound healing it is not a common cause for skin graft failure. Skin grafts applied to well vascularised beds fail because of haematoma or seroma formation, infection, mechanical shear or technical errors such as erroneously placing the graft upside down.

6.8
Answer D
Each osteon comprises of osteocytes and a central haversian canal that contains a nutrient vessel. Osteons are connected to each other by tranverse nutrient canals knowm as Volkmann's canals.

6.9
Answer C
Melanin is the chromophore used in hair removal.

6.10
Answer C

6.11
Answer D
Rectangular shaped expanders produce the greatest gain in expanded tissue area.

6.12
Answer D
Treacher Collins presents with a combination of Tessier clefts 6, 7 and 8.

6.13
Answer A
Romberg's hemifacial atrophy usually presents after 5 years of age (usually in the early teen years). It is progressive and the disease usually 'burns out' in the mid-twenties. It is not associated with a positive family history and occurs sporadically. It is thought to be due to a viral infection or an abnormality of the sympathetic nervous system. It presents with progreesive, localised atrophy of the soft tissues of the face and may involve the underlying skeleton. It may present with a sharp depression of the forehead known as the 'coup de sabre'.

6.14
Answer B
The most common form of synostosis involves premature fusion of the sagittal suture. This accounts for half of all cranial synostoses.

6.15
Answer B
In' true' plagiocephaly the skull is shaped like a rhomboid (or parallelogram) whereas in 'positional' plagiocephaly the skull is shaped like a triangle with its apex lying on the affected side.

6.16
Answer D
Allografts refer to non-living tissue derived from the same species eg. Cadaveric skin.

6.17
Answer C
Isolated cleft palate differs from cleft lip and palate in that it is more common in females, more likely to be associated with a syndrome and less associated with familial factors.

6.18
Answer B
Complete cleft lip is associated with a degree of nasal deformity. There is a decrease in the vertical height of the lip because of a soft tissue deficiency, abnormal insertion of the muscles, a cleft in the alveolus and defect of the hard palate anterior to the incisive foramen.

6.19
Answer C
The primary problem that intiates the Pierre-Robin sequence is a small jaw.

6.20
Answer C
Giant congenital hairy naevii are not confined to the dermis and may invade underlying structures. There is a 5 – 10% risk of malignant transformation.

6.21
Answer A
Basal cell carcinoma is the most common form of skin cancer.

6.22
Answer A
All BCC's arise from the pluripotential cells of the epidermis at the dermoepidermal junction.

6.23
Answer C
Keratoacanthomas demonstrate rapid growth and are known to resolve spontaneously. Ferguson-Smith syndrome is an autosomal dominant condition that presents with multiple self-healing epitheliomas. Keratoacanthomas are difficult to differentiate from squamous cell carcinomas clinically and even histologically.

6.24
Answer B
Broder's classification is based on histological analysis and is denoted by the ratio of differentiated to undifferentiated cells.
Grade 1: 3 : 1
Grade 2: 1 : 1
Grade 3: 1 : 3
Grade 4: Tumour has no tendency towards differentiation

6.25
Answer C
A tumour extending to the junction of the papillary and reticular dermis corresponds to Clark's level 3. It is not possible to determine the Breslow thickness from the information provided in the stem of the question. In an non-ulcerated lesion the Breslow thickness of the tumour is measured from the granular layer to the maximum depth of the tumour.

6.26
Answer C
Despite the tendency to blame the anaesthetist sometimes, and although this does sometimes bring some degree of self-satisfaction and comfort, this problem is not due to an anaesthetic problem but is typical of the 'no-reflow' phenomenon. The vessels are patent and therefore it is unlikely to arise secondary to a technical problem.

6.27
Answer D
Heparin inhibits thrombin and factor Xa by binding to antithrombin III. Aspirin acts by inhibiting platelet aggregation through the inhibition of cyclooxygenase.

6.28
Answer C
The rib cartilages used in total ear reconstruction are only large enough in children 6 years of age to create an adult size ear.

6.29
Answer D
T1-weighted images – fat appear white
T2-weighted images – water appear white
T2-weighted images are useful for demonstrating areas of inflammation within tissues.

6.30
Answer A
Adenoid cystic carcinoma is well known for perineural invasion of the facial nerve and for producing skip lesions along the nerve. It is a difficult tumour to eradicate and it has a high rate of recurrence.

6.31
Answer B
This patient is not suitable for any complex microsurgical procedures and therefore the most appropriate option is a bridging contoured plate and coverage of the metal work with locally available soft tissues.

6.32
Answer D
The facial nerve provides motor innervation to the muscles of facial expression.

6.33
Answer C
In this case the function of the frontalis muscle is intact on the affected side. Hence, this is a lower motor neurone lesion distal to the nucleus of the facial nerve. The nerve to the stapedius muscle is involved (hence the hyperacusis). This is an intratemporal branch of the facial nerve. Hence, this lesion is most certainly intratemporal.

157

6.34
Answer B
The muscles of facial expression are a second branchial arch derivative. The first branchial arch gives rise to the maxilla, mandible and muscles of mastication.

6.35
Answer C
The stylopharyngeus muscle is a derivative of the third branchial arch and is innervated by the glossopharyngeal nerve (CN IX).

6.36
Answer A
The internal mammary artery is the dominant blood supply to the breast. The breast also receives a blood supply from the lateral thoracic artery, highest thoracic artery and the lateral branches of the 3rd, 4th and 5th posterior intercostals arteries.

6.37
Answer B
The most appropriate method of reconstruction here considering that the patient has not undergone radiotherapy and that she is slim and athletic would be the insertion of an expander initially followed by its replacement for a definitive implant after adequate expansion.

6.38
Answer A
The soleus muscle flap is appropriate for the coverage of defects of the middle third of the leg. The medial or lateral heads of the gastrocnemius muscle maybe used depending on the location and extent of the defect. In general, the medial head of the gastrocnemius muscle is used more frequently since it tends to be slightly longer than the lateral head.

6.39
Answer A
Botulinum toxin has been licensed for the treatment of blepharospasm, hemifacial spasm, cervical dystonia, severe hyperhidrosis of the axillae, dynamic equines foot deformity due to spasticity in ambulant paediatric (2 years or older) patients with cerebral palsy and for glabella lines.

6.40
Answer B
Obstruction of the visual axis for a week or more in the first year of life can result in deprivation amblyopia and anisotropia. Therefore any lesion present in the periocular region which can potentially obstruct vision should be treated. Haemangiomas naturally increase in size in the first year of life. This by itself is not an indication for treatment since most will spontaneously involute. However, if it causes significant obstruction of the vision axis, auditory canal or upper respiratory tract; or if it causes ulceration and bleeding then it should be treated and not left to spontaneously involute.

6.41
Answer B

6.42
Answer F

6.43
Answer C

6.44
Answer D

6.45
Answer K

6.46
Answer F

6.47
Answer C

6.48
Answer A

6.49
Answer D

6.50
Answer H

QUIZ 7
MULTIPLE CHOICE QUESTIONS

For questions 7.1 to 7.40 please the ONE most appropriate answer.

Q 7.1
Which of the following is a feature of apocrine sweat glands?

[A] Mostly found on the palm of the hand and sole of the foot

[B] Secrete ruptured vesicles via the process of exocytosis

[C] Secrete whole cells

[D] Mainly located in the axilla and groin

Q 7.2

The extended area of skin which is perfused by a named artery after a delaying procedure is known as the

[A] Anatomical territory of the artery

[B] Dynamic territory of the artery

[C] Potential territory of the artery

[D] Choke area of the artery

Q 7.3
Which of the following is not essential for wound healing?

[A] Vitamin A

[B] Vitamin C

[C] Vitamin D

[D] Vitamin E

Q 7.4
A new Class IV Nd:YAG laser is available for use in your department. Which of the following statements is TRUE?

[A] Lasers are rated by their potential to induce ocular damage

[B] Lasers are rated by their depth of penetrance of solid lead shields

[C] The smoke fumes generated by the use of lasers are not as hazardous as that produced by electrocautery

[D] Flammable liquids can be safely used with lasers since the heat produced is deep within the tissues

Q 7.5
Which of the following is NOT recognised stage of process of wound epithelialisation?

[A] Migration

[B] Inosculation

[C] Mobilisation

[D] Cellular mitosis and differentiation

Q 7.6
Which one of the following dressings contains cultured cells?

[A] Transcyte

[B] Integra

[C] Alloderm

[D] Biobrane

Q 7.7
Which one of the following statements about sutures is TRUE?

[A] Wound infection prolongs suture absorption

[B] Polyglactin is absorbed through a proteolytic process

[C] Poliglecaprone is absorbed through a hydrolytic process

[D] Knot security is directly proportional to the coefficient of friction of the suture material

Q 7.8
A tissue expander is being inserted under the scalp for the reconstruction of a skin grafted area of 7 x 7cm. Ideally, where should the incision be made for the insertion of the expander?

[A] Along the edge of the skin graft

[B] A W-shaped incision within the skin grafted area

[C] A radial incision outside of the skin grafted area

[D] An incision parallel to the edge of the skin a distance equal to one diameter away from the edge of the skin graft

Q 7.9
Which of the following is NOT a feature of Treacher Collins syndrome?

[A] It is unilateral combination of Tessier clefts nos. 6 - 8

[B] Colobomas

[C] Downward slanting of the eyes laterally

[D] Microtia

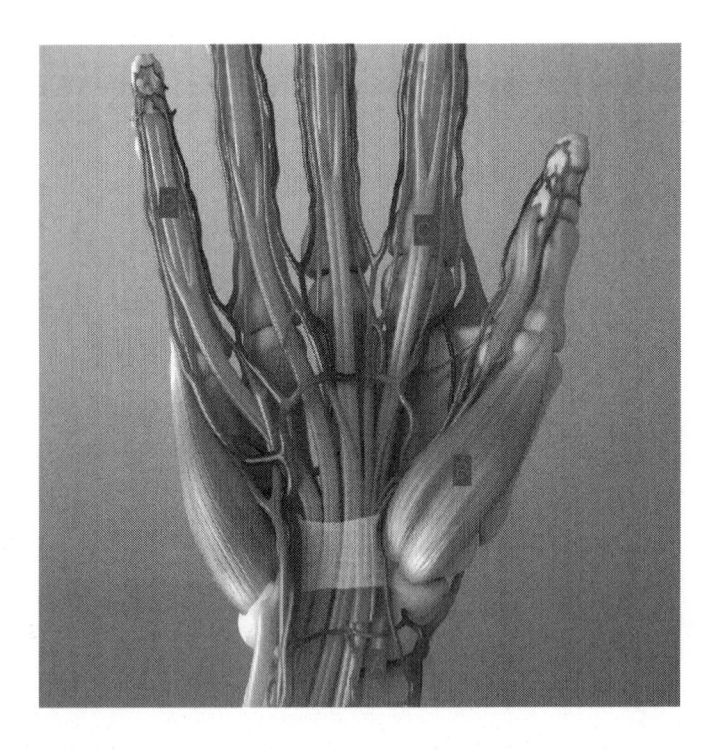

Q 7.10
Which of the following annotated structures in the figure of the hand above corresponds to the flexor pollicis longus?

Q 7.11
Cranial growth in infancy occurs as a response to which of the following?

[A] Brain growth

[B] Premature fusion of the cranial sutures

[C] A steady independent deposition of bone

[D] Good nutrition

Q 7.12
Which of the following is NOT a characteristic feature of the nasal deformity associated with a cleft lip?

[A] A kink of the lateral crus of the lower alar cartilage on the contralateral side

[B] Separation of the domes of the alar cartilages at the tip of the nose

[C] Retrodisplacement of the nasal base on the ipsilateral side

[D] Deviation of the nasal spine away from the cleft side

Q 7.13
With regards to cleft lip and palate repair, which of the following statements is TRUE?

[A] The cleft lip component should be repaired in the first 48 hours after birth to prevent long term scarring and deformity

[B] The cleft palate component should be repaired in the first 48 hours to prevent disturbance of midfacial growth in the first year of life

[C] Presurgical orthopaedics is mandatory in the first 48 hours of life

[D] The Schweckendiek technique recommends hard palatal repair at approximately 8 years of age

Q 7.14
A 65 year-old gentleman had a basal cell carcinoma completely excised from left cheek 6 weeks ago. What is the risk of him having a new primary BCC within the next 5 years?

[A] <10%

[B] 15%

[C] 50%

[D] 85%

Q 7.15
With regards to primary cutaneous SCC's, which one of the following statements is TRUE?

[A] There is a clear role for sentinel lymph node biopsy in the treatment protocol

[B] Immunosuppresed patients do not have an increased risk of metastasis

[C] Moh's surgery is not a treatment modality since this is only applicable to BCC's

[D] Ninety-five percent of local recurrences and metastases are detected in the first 5 years following treatment

Q 7.16
By definition, the Breslow thickness of a non-ulcerated malignant melanoma is the measure of the thickness of the tumour measured from which of the following cellular areas?

[A] Basal layer

[B] Stratum spinosum

[C] Stratum granulosum

[D] Stratum corneum

Q 7.17
A 57 year gentleman has had a 2.1cm well-differentiated SCC excised from the left lower leg? What is the likely overall risk of this patient developing metastasis?

[A] 9%

[B] 15%

[C] 23%

[D] 30%

Q 7.18
Which of the following most accurately outlines the mechanism of action of heparin?

[A] Inhibits platelet aggregation through the inhibition of cyclooxygenase

[B] Inactivates Von Willebrand factor

[C] Increases the number of mast cells

[D] Inhibits thrombin and factor Xa by binding to antithrombin III

Q 7.19
What proportion of Caucasians undergoing bilateral prominent ear correction develops postauricular hypertrophic scars?

[A] 3%

[B] 6%

[C] 10%

[D] 20%

Q 7.20
A 59 year-old man underwent a right superficial parotidectomy 1 year ago. He is now experiencing sweating in the region of the right ear and temple everytime he having a meal. What is the pathophysiology of his condition?

[A] Reinnervation of the sympathetic sweat glands along the distribution of innervation of the auriculotemporal nerve by regenerated postganglionic parasympathetic nerve fibres

[B] Reinnervation of the parasympathetic sweat glands along the distribution of innervation of the auriculotemporal nerve by regenerated postganglionic sympathetic nerve fibres

[C] Reinnervation of the parasympathetic sweat glands along the distribution of innervation of the auriculotemporal nerve by regenerated preganglionic sympathetic nerve fibres

[D] Reinnervation of the sympathetic sweat glands along the distribution of innervation of the facial nerve by regenerated postganglionic sympathetic nerve fibres

Q 7.21
Which of the following is NOT a recognised treatment of Frey's syndrome?

[A] Botulinum toxin injection

[B] Amitriptylline

[C] Antiperspirants

[D] Dermofat grafts

Q 7.22
How does a positron emission scan work?

[A] Uses strong magnetic waves

[B] Uses sound waves

[C] Depends on increased uptake of radioactive 8-fluorodeoxyglucose by tissues with high metabolic rates

[D] Depends on increased uptake of radioactive 18-fluorodeoxyglucose by tissues with high metabolic rates

Q 7.23
Which of the following does NOT contribute to the blood supply of the nose?

[A] Branches of the ophthalmic artery

[B] Supratrochlear artery

[C] Greater palatine artery

[D] Superior labial artery

Q 7.24
Which of the following signs is indicative of a parotid tumour infiltrating into the facial nerve?

[A] Hyperacusis

[B] Altered sensation over the forehead on the ipsilateral side

[C] Drooling from the corner of the mouth on the ipsilateral side

[D] Loss of taste to the anterior two-thirds of the tongue

Q 7.25
Which of the following nerves provides the primary innervation of the nipple?

[A] Supraclavicular nerves

[B] Anterior branch of the 2nd intercostal nerve

[C] Lateral cutaneous branch of the T4

[D] Anterior branch of the 3rd intercostals nerve

Q 7.26
Which of the following statements regarding tamoxifen is TRUE?

[A] It marginally reduces the chance of developing breast cancer in women of increased risk

[B] It is more beneficial in women who have oestrogen-negative tumours

[C] It is only useful in premonopausal women

[D] Maybe used to treat infertility in women with anovulatory cycles

Q 7.27
Which of the following signs is NOT suspicious for breast cancer on mammography?

[A] The Linguine sign

[B] Speckled microcalcifications

[C] Architectural distortion

[D] Asymmetry

Q 7.28
Which of the following drugs is NOT regarded as a cause of gynaecomastia?

[A] Amoxicillin

[B] Metronidazole

[C] Enalapril

[D] Marijuana

Q 7.29
A 23 year old patient sustains a severe dog bite injury to the area just distal to the medial malleolus of the left leg. After an debridement the patient is left with a defect which is 5cm in diameter with exposed bone stripped of periosteum. The injury is isolated to the medial ankle. Which of the following form of reconstruction would be most appropriate for this patient?

[A] Topical negative pressure therapy

[B] Topical negative pressure therapy followed by a split-thickness skin graft once the wound has sufficiently granulated and wound swabs of the wound are negative

[C] A distally based medial gastrocnemius muscle flap

[D] A reverse flow adipofascial sural artery neurocutaneous flap with a split-thickness skin graft

Q 7.30
Which of the following statements concerning hypospadias is TRUE?

[A] About 50% of cases are associated with inguinal hernias

[B] About 50% of cases are associated with undescended testes

[C] Undescended testes may indicate an intersex state

[D] Most cases of hypospadias are proximal

Q 7.31
Which of the following statements is TRUE in relation to Poland's syndrome?

[A] It is more common in females

[B] It is more common on the left side

[C] It is associated with a genetic link

[D] It is thought to arise from a kinking of the subclavian artery during embryological development

Q 7.32
Which of the following entities refer to a true haemangioma?

[A] Strawberry naevus

[B] Cavernous haemangioma

[C] Salmon patch

[D] Port wine stain

Q 7.33
Which of the following is characteristic of the endothelium of a haemangioma?

[A] The endothelial cells are narrow and have a 'picket-fence' pattern of arrangement

[B] There is an increase in number of macrophages between the endothelial cells

[C] The endothelial cells have a longer lifespan than the normal

[D] There is an increase in the number of mast cells

Q 7.34
Which ONE of the following chemical peeling agents can be used for a medium-depth peel?

[A] Phenol

[B] Trichloroacetic acid (TCA)

[C] Glycolic acid

[D] Salicylic acid

Q 7.35
Which ONE of the following is NOT example of a vascular malformation?

[A] Port-wine stain

[B] Lymphatic malformation

[C] Haemangioma

[D] Venular malformation

Q 7.36
Which ONE of the following is NOT a true retaining ligament of the face?

[A] Zygomatic ligament

[B] Masseteric ligament

[C] Lateral orbital thickening

[D] Mandibular retaining ligament

173

Q 7.37
How many fat compartments are there in the upper eyelids?

[A] 1

[B] 2

[C] 3

[D] 4

Q 7.38
Which of the following structures is located between the middle and nasal fat pads of the upper eyelid?

[A] The trochlear of the inferior oblique muscle

[B] The medial rectus muscle

[C] The lateral rectus muscle

[D] The trochlear of the superior oblique muscle

Q 7.39
Which of the following is NOT a function of the superior oblique muscle in relation to eyeball movement?

[A] Oblique rotation

[B] Internal rotation

[C] Depression

[D] Lateral rotation

Q 7.40
What is the blood loss with tumescent liposuction?

[A] 1-7%

[B] 15-30%

[C] 20-25%

[D] 20-45%

QUIZ 7

EXTENDED MATCHING QUESTIONS

For questions 7.41 to 7.45 please select the ONE MOST appropriate answer from list [A] to [K]. Each answer maybe used more than once or not at all.

The following is a list of blood vessels relating to free flaps.

[A] Thoracodorsal vessels
[B] Superficial temporal vessels
[C] Descending branch of the circumflex scapular vessels
[D] Subscapular vessels
[E] Ascending branch of the lateral circumflex femoral vessels
[F] Descending branch of the lateral circumflex femoral vessels
[G] Transverse cervical vessels
[H] Medial circumflex femoral vessels
[J] Superficial circumflex iliac vessels
[K] Deep circumflex iliac vessels

Which one of the above blood vessel match most closely to the blood supply of the following free flaps?

Q 7.41
Groin flap

Q 7.42
Tensor fascia lata flap

Q 7.43
Gracilis flap

Q7.44
Parascapular flap

Q 7.45
Anterolateral flap

For questions 7.46 to 7.50 please select the ONE MOST appropriate answer from list [A] to [K]. Each answer maybe used more than once or not at all.

The following is a list of bones of the hand and wrist.

[A] Scaphoid
[B] Trapezium
[C] Lunate
[D] Hamate
[E] Trapezoid
[F] Capitate
[G] Pisiform
[H] Triquetrum
[J] Head of ulnar
[K] Styloid process of ulnar

Please identify the following stuctures which are labeled on the figure below.

Q 7.46
91

Q 7.47
92

Q 7.48
93

Q 7.49
94

Q 7.50
95

178

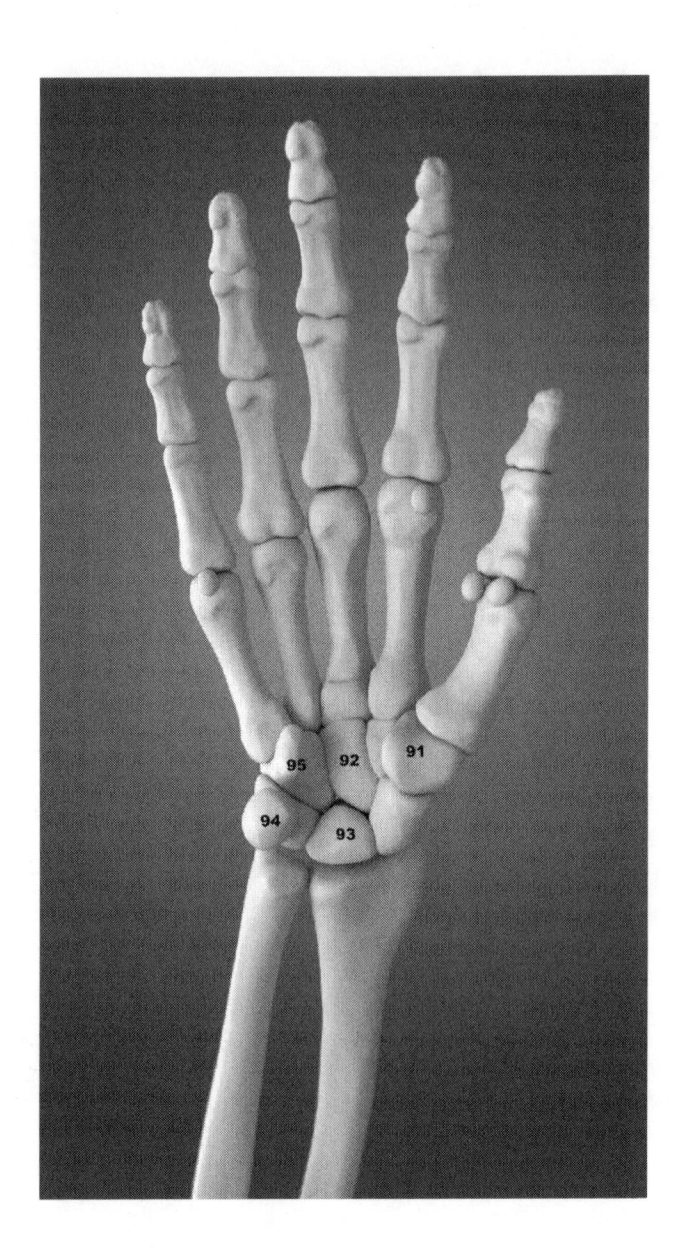

QUIZ 7
ANSWERS

7.1
Answer D
Apocrine sweat glands are mainly located in the axilla and groin. They secrete unruptured vesicles. Infection involving these glands result in hidradenitis suppurativa.

7.2
Answer C
The potential territory of a named artery is the extended area of skin that is supplied by the artery after undergoing a delaying procedure.

7.3
Answer C
Deficiencies of vitamins A, C and E result in poor wound healing. Vitamin C is required for collagen synthesis and vitamin E is a membrane stabilizer. Vitamin D is important in calcium metabolism.

7.4
Answer A
Lasers are rated by their potential to induce ocular damage. Because the smoke fumes may contain traces of blood and potentially viruses, special laser quality masks must be worn. Flammable prep must not be used.

7.5
Answer B

The stages of wound epithelialisation are mobilisation (initiated by the loss of contact inhibition), migration, cellular mitosis and differentiation. Inosculation is one of the mechanisms of revascularisation of a skin graft during the 'graft take' process. This process involves the direct spontaneous anastomosis between the vessels of the graft with those on the recipient bed.

7.6
Answer A

Transcyte consists of neonatal fibroblasts seeded onto a silicone/collagen matrix and covered a nylon sheet. Biobrane is is a nylon sheet covering a silicone layer containing dermal collagen. Integra is a bilaminar sheet consisting of silicone covering an artificial dermis made with bovine collagen and glycosaminoglycanss from shark. Alloderm is de-epithelialised acellular cadaveric skin.

Split-thickness skin grafts have less dermal elements than full-thickness grafts. As a result there is less primary contraction and greater secondary contraction than full-thickness grafts.

7.7
Answer C

Wound infection speeds up the rate of suture absorption. Synthetic absorbable sutures are absorbed by a process of hydrolysis whereby natural absorbable sutures are absorbed by a proteolytic process.

7.8
Answer B

Ideally the incision should be within the skin graft since this is expected to be excised anyway. An incision along the margin of the skin graft may have an increased risk of implant extrusion. Any incision away from the skin graft within the normal tissue may compromise the perfusion of the expander skin flap.

7.9
Answer A
Treacher Collins syndrome is an autosomal dominant bilateral confluent Tessier clefts 6 – 8.

7.10
Answer A

7.11
Answer A
Normal cranial growth responds to increased brain volume.

7.12
Answer A
The features of the nasal deformity associates with a cleft lip are:
- Deviation of the nasal spine away from the cleft side
- A kink of the lateral crus of the lower alar cartilage on the *cleft* side
- Separation of the domes of the alar cartilages at the tip of the nose
- Retrodisplacement of the nasal base on the ipsilateral side
- Dislocation of the upper lateral cartilage from the lower lateral cartilage on the cleft side
- Flattening and displacement of the nasal bone on the cleft side

7.13
Answer D
With the Schweckendiek technique the lip and soft palate are repaired before 1 year of age and hard palate is repaired at about 8 years of age.

7.14
Answer C
In a patient with a completely excised primary Bcc, the risk of a new primary is 35% at 3 years and 50% at 5 years.

7.15
Answer D
There is no clear role for sentinel lymph node biopsy in the treatment protocol of SCC's. Immunosuppressed patients have a higher risk of metastasis. Moh's surgery is particularly useful in the treatment of high-risk SCC's, recurrent SCC's and SCC's in area of cosmetic importance. Ninety-five percent of local recurrences and metastases are detected in the first 5 years following treatment.

7.16
Answer C
The Breslow thickness is measured from the granular layer in non-ulcerated lesions and from the base of ulcer in ulcerated lesions.

7.17
Answer A
The risk of a patient with a well-differentiated T2 lesion developing metastases is 7-9%.

7.18
Answer D
Heparin inhibits thrombin and factor Xa by binding to antithrombin III. Aspirin acts by inhibiting platelet aggregation through the inhibition of cyclooxygenase.

7.19
Answer A
There is about a 3% risk of hypertrophic scar formation in Caucasian children undergoing bilateral prominent ear correction.

7.20
Answer A
This is known as Frey's syndrome. Postganglionic parasympathetic nerve fibres destined for the parotid gland get there by hitch-hiking on the auriculotemporal nerve. During parotidectomy these fibres are divided. These fibres first degenerate to the level of the cell bodies in the otic ganglion and then regenerate again, hitch-hiking on the auriculotemporal nerve. Since the target organ has been removed they then go on to connect to the sympathetic sweat glands. Therefore, eating triggers profuse sweating in the distribution of the auriculotemporal nerve.

7.21
Answer B
Antiperspirant use, botulinum toxin A, surgical transaction of the nerve fibres and interpositional dermofat grafts are recognised modes of treatment for Frey's syndrome.

7.22
Answer D
Positron emission scans depends on the increased uptake of 18-fluorodeoxyglucose by tissues with high metabolic rates (such as tumours).

7.23
Answer B
The arterial supply to the nose includes branches from the internal carotid (the branches of the anterior and posterior ethmoid arteries from the ophthalmic artery) and branches from the external carotid (sphenopalatine, greater palatine, superior labial, and angular arteries).

7.24
Answer C
The facial nerve branches within the substance of the parotid gland into five branches to innervate the muscles of facial expression.

183

7.25
Answer C
The nipple is innervated by the lateral cutaneous branch of T4.

7.26
Answer D
Tamoxifen can reduce the chance of developing breast cancer in high risk women quite significantly. It is more beneficial in women who have oestrogen-positive tumours. It maybe used to treat infertility in women with anovulatory cycles.

7.27
Answer A
The signs which are suspicious of breast cancer on mammography are speckled microcalcifications, density changes, asymmetry and architectural distortion of the breast tissues.
The Linguine sign is diagnostic of an intracapsular rupture of a silicone breast implant on a T2-weighted MRI scan.

7.28
Answer A
Metronidazole, enalapril and marijuana are all known to cause gynaecomastia.

7.29
Answer D
This is the case of a young patient with defect of the medial ankle with exposed bone stripped of periosteum at the base. This defect should be reconstructed as soon as the wound has been adequately debrided and is free of pathogens. Therefore, topical negative pressure therapy is ideally not an appropriate form of treatment for this defect. Although, the distally based gastocnemius muscle flap has been described for the coverage of defects of the distal third of the leg in war injuries, this defect is too distal for its consideration. The zone of injury is confined to the medial ankle and hence the lateral perforator which facilitates the reverse flow to the sural artery neurocutaneous flap should be intact in this patient and this makes it an attractive option.

7.30
Answer C
Hypospadias with undescended testes may indicate an intersex state. About 9% of cases of hypospadias present with inguinal hernias and a similar proportion of cases with undescended testes. These increase with more proximal hypospadias.

7.31
Answer D
Poland's syndrome is mostly sporadic and is thought to arise from the kinking of the subclavian artery at around the 6th week of gestation. It is equally common in males and females and more common on the right side.

7.32
Answer A
Some haemangiomas are commonly referred to strawberry naevii. A cavernous haemangioma is venous vascular malformation. A port wine stain is a capillary haemangioma.

7.33
Answer D
Histologically, haemangiomas consist of plump, hyperplastic endothelial cells which have a rapid turnover rate. There is an increase in the number of mast cells.

7.34
Answer B
Glycolic and salicyclic acids are used for superficial peels whereas, phenols are used for deep peels.

7.35
Answer C
Port-wine stains, venous ,venular, arterial, arterio-venous and lymphativ malformations are all vascular malformations. Haemangiomas, telangiectasia and spider angiomas are not.

7.36
Answer B
True retaining ligaments are easily identifiable and connect the dermis to the underlying periosteum. The zygomatic ligament, lateral orbital thickening and the mandibular ligaments are true retaining ligaments. False retaining ligaments are more diffuse and connect the superficial and deep facial fascia. The masseteric ligament is a false retaining ligament of the cheek.

7.37
Answer B
There are 2 fat compartments in the upper eyelid.

7.38
Answer D
The trochlear of the superior oblique muscle lies between the middle and nasal fat pads of the upper eyelid. It maybe damaged during blepharoplasty.

7.39
Answer A
The primary action of the superior oblique muscle is internal rotation of the eyeball. The secondary action is depression and the tertiary action is lateral rotation.

7.40
Answer A
The blood loss with the tumescent technique is between 1-7%.

7.41
Answer J

7.42
Answer E

7.43
Answer H

7.44
Answer C

7.45
Answer F

7.46
Answer B

7.47
Answer E

7.48
Answer C

7.49
Answer G

7.50
Answer D

QUIZ 8
MULTIPLE CHOICE QUESTIONS

For questions 8.1 to 8.40 please the ONE most appropriate answer.

Q 8.1

What proportion of haemangiomas is expected to spontaneously resolve at 7 years of age?

[A] 40%

[B] 50%

[C] 60%

[D] 70%

Q 8.2
Which is the following is most likely location of the inferior oblique muscle?

[A] Medial to the nasal fat pad

[B] Between the middle and medial fat pads

[C] Between the lateral and middle fat pads

[D] Lateral to the lateral fat pad

Q 8.3
Which of the following nerves innervate the inferior oblique muscle?

[A] Optic nerve

[B] Oculomotor nerve

[C] Trochlear nerve

[D] Abducens nerve

Q 8.4
You are called to the neonatal unit to see a 5-hour old infant with a hugh bluish lesion occupying most of the anterior and lateral aspects of the right thigh. You are told than the neonate is severely thrombopenic with an abnormal clotting screen, reduced fibrinogen levels and elevated levels of fibrin degradation products. What is the most likely diagnosis?

[A] Severe sickle cell anaemia

[B] Haemangioendothelioma

[C] Large arteriovenous malformation

[D] Idiopathic thrombocytopenia

Q 8.5
What is the normal inter-orbital distance?

[A] 23 – 28mm

[B] 30 – 34mm

[C] 35 – 39mm

[D] 40 – 45mm

Q 8.6
A 20 year-old patient presents with an open fracture of the left tibia with a 10cm gaping wound on the anterior aspect of the left leg. He is taken to theatre within 6 hours and the wound is adequately debrided left open and also undergoes internal fixation of the fractured tibia. Five hours post-operatively he complains of severe pain in the limb. A diagnosis of compartment syndrome is arrived at and he taken to theatre for fasciotomy. How many compartments need to be decompressed in this patient?

[A] 2

[B] 3

[C] 4

[D] 5

Q 8.7
Which of the following statements MOST accurately describes a subcutaneous mastectomy?

[A] Excision of all of the breast tissue and the overlying skin

[B] Excision of the breast tissue preserving the overlying skin

[C] Excision of most of the breast tissue preserving the nipple-areolar complex and overlying skin

[D] Excision of the breast and nipple-areolar complex and preserving the overlying skin flaps

Q 8.8
A patient undergoing a delayed DIEP flap breast reconstruction is more likely to experience which one of the following complications compared to undergoing a free TRAM flap breast reconstruction?

[A] Abdominal bulge

[B] Fat necrosis

[C] Flap failure

[D] Decreased function of the rectus abdominis

Q 8.9
A 26 year old male student presents to you with increased breast size. He says that he developed this since he was 14 years of age and it has not reduced in size since. On examination both breasts are symmetrical and moderately enlarged with noticeable skin excess and mild ptosis. What grade would this fall under in the Simon's classification of gynaecomastia?

[A] Grade 1

[B] Grade 2

[C] Grade 2B

[D] Grade

Q 8.10
The external auditory canal is a derivative of the following embryological structures?

[A] The first branchial arch

[B] The fist branchial cleft

[C] The second branchial arch

[D] The second branchial cleft

Q 8.11
Acetylcholine is the neurotransmitter which is present between the pre- and ganglionic fibres of the facial nerve. Acetylcholine is attaches to which of the following receptors?

[A] Nicotinic

[B] Dopaminergic

[C] GABAergic

[D] Histaminergic

Q 8.12
Branches of the facial nerve innervate the muscles of facial expression. It enters the following muscles on their superficial surface except?

[A] Mentalis

[B] Buccinator

[C] Levator anguli superioris

[D] Depressor naguli oris

Q 8.13
What is the innervation of Müller's muscle?

[A] The oculomotor nerve

[B] The trochlear nerve

[C] Parasympathetic fibres

[D] Sympathetic fibres

Q 8.14
What is the MOST common skin malignancy of the lower eyelid?

[A] Basal cell carcinoma

[B] Squamous cell carcinoma

[C] Porocarcinoma

[D] Merkel cell tumour

Q 8.15
What is the normal chondromastoid angle in an average adult?

[A] 5°

[B] 106°

[C] 31°

[D] 47°

Q 8.16
Performing microsurgery in patients who smoke does is usually a cause of uneasiness. Which of the following statements is TRUE?

[A] Smoking after a digital replant results in a high failure rate

[B] There is a higher rate of free flap failure in smokers

[C] Smoking is an absolute contraindication in patients who smoke

[D] There is no increase in wound healing complications in smokers undergoing microsurgery

Q 8.17
Which of the following statements regarding Dextran 40 is correct?

[A] It is a glycosaminoglycan

[B] It inactivates von Willebrand's factor

[C] It is routinely used in microsurgery

[D] It is non-allergenic

Q 8.18
The Trojani classification of soft tissue sarcomas involves all of the following parameters EXCEPT?

[A] Size of the lesion

[B] Degree of necrosis

[C] Degree of differentiation

[D] Mitotic index

Q 8.19
The histology report for a patient with a malignant melanoma of the right anterior chest wall indicated that the tumour extended to junction of the papillary and reticular dermis. This corresponds to which of the following?

[A] At least a Breslow thickness of 2.0mm

[B] At least a Breslow thickness of 1.0 mm

[C] Clark's level 3

[D] Clark's level

Q 8.20
Which of the following statements regarding sentinel lymph node biopsy is correct?

[A] It is only useful in the treatment of malignant melanoma

[B] It is now mandatory for the treatment of all malignant melanoma

[C] It has been shown to confer a disease-free survival benefit in patients with intermediate-thickness primary melanomas

[D] It has no role in the staging of the disease

Q 8.21
Basal cell carcinomas occur most commonly on?

[A] Trunk

[B] Upper limbs

[C] Lower limbs

[D] Head and neck regions

Q 8.22
What proportion of patients with cleft lip and palate have an isolated cleft palate?

[A] 10%

[B] 30%

[C] 50%

[D] 60%

Q 8.23
What is the primary abnormality that results in the Pierre-Robin sequence?

[A] Failure of rotation of the palatal shelves

[B] Failure of the tongue to descend

[C] A small jaw

[D] Failure of fusion of the palatal shelves resulting in a U-shaped cleft palate

Q 8.24
Which of the following factors would adverse affect the survival of a non-vascularised bone graft?

[A] Bone graft with an intact periosteum

[B] A bone graft placed in an orthotopic position

[C] A bone graft placed in a heterotopic position

[D] A rigidly fixed bone graft

Q 8.25
Which of the following statements is TRUE of Alloderm®?

[A] It is derived from the skin of pigs

[B] It is a permanent skin substitute

[C] It is highly allergenic

[D] It is acellular human cadaveric dermis

Q 8.26
All of the following are clinical features of true plagiocephaly EXCEPT?

[A] The skull is triangular shaped

[B] Prominence of the ipsilateral cheek

[C] The distance between the lateral orbit and the ear is decreased on the ipsilateral side

[D] Prominence of the contralateral brow

Q 8.27
Which of the following is NOT a feature of Treacher Collins syndrome?

[A] It is unilateral combination of Tessier clefts nos. 6 - 8

[B] Colobomas

[C] Downward slanting of the eyes laterally

[D] Microtia

Q 8.28
A 3-month old infant presents to the outpatient clinic with a left sided microtia. On further evaluation she is also noted to have left midface hypolasia. Which of the following is the MOST LIKELY diagnosis?

[A] Treacher Collins syndrome

[B] Romberg's hemifacial atrophy

[C] Left hemifacial microsomia

[D] Mobeius syndrome

Q 8.29
The gain in the area of tissue obtained through expansion is influenced by the shape of the expander. Which of the following shapes of expanders produces the maximal gain in surface area of the expanded skin?

[A] Round

[B] Oval

[C] Crescentic

[D] Rectangular

Q 8.30
Lasers use the technique of selective photothermolysis. What is the chromophore for the Nd:YAG laser when used for hair removal?

[A] Water

[B] Haemoglobin

[C] Melanin

[D] Collagen

Q 8.31
What is the mechanism of action of intralesional steroids in the treatment of hypertrophic scarring?

[A] Inhibits collagenase production

[B] Inhibits fibroblast proliferation

[C] Induces an inflammatory reaction in the scar

[D] Increases collagen production

Q 8.32
What species of bacteria are found in the gut of leeches?

[A] *Eikenella corrodens*

[B] *Staphylococcus aureus*

[C] *Pasturella moltocida*

[D] *Aeromonas hydrophilia*

Q 8.33
With regards to the structure of cortical bone, each individual bone unit called an osteon comprises all of the following EXCEPT?

[A] Osteocytes

[B] A central nutrient blood vessel

[C] A haversian canal

[D] A Volkmann's canal

Q 8.34

A 72 year old gentleman had an excision of an SCC from his frontal scalp. The resultant defect was partially devoid of periosteum. He underwent reconstruction of the defect using a rotation flap and subsequently, the flap was re-elevated in a more superficial plane and replaced in its original location. Theoriginal defect is now graftable. What is the term used to describe this principle?

[A] Virchow's principle

[B] Moss's principle

[C] Crane principle

[D] Von Langenbeck's principle

199

Q 8.35

In which of the following patients it would be safe to perform an elective facelift procedure?

[A] A patient with cutis laxa

[B] A patient with progeria

[C] A patient with Ehlers-Danlos syndrome

[D] None of the above

Q 8.36
Vacuum-assisted wound closure work using the following techniques EXCEPT?

[A] Increases the rate of granulation tissue formation

[B] Direct suction on the wound edges result in wound contraction

[C] Decreases the bacterial load of the wound

[D] Increases the concentration of tissue metalloproteinases in the wound

Q 8.37
Which of the following is the best description of a reverse-cutting needle?

[A] They have a flat surface on the inner side of the curve of the needle

[B] They have a sharp edge on the inner side of the curve of the needle

[C] They have a sharp tip but no sharp edge

[D] They are not as sharp as conventional cutting needles

Q 8.38
What is the most common site of cervical metastasis of a squamous cell carcinoma of the anterior two-thirds of the tongue?

[A] Level I lymph node

[B] Level II lymph node

[C] Level III lymph node

[D] Lungs

Q 8.39
Where does the facial nerve lies in relation to the tragal pointer?

[A] 1cm deep and 1cm inferior to the tragal pointer

[B] 1cm deep and 1cm superior to the tragal pointer

[C] 1cm superficial and 1cm inferior to the tragal pointer

[D] 1cm superficial and 1cm superior to the tragal pointer

Q 8.40
Which of the following statements about TRAM flap breast reconstruction is FALSE?

[A] The superior epigastric artery is the dominant vascular axis

[B] It is a Type II myocutaneous flap based on the Mathes and Nahai classification

[C] It is regarded as a type of autologous breast reconstruction

[D] A delay procedure involving ligation of the deep inferior epigastric vessels 2-3 weeks prior to a pedicle TRAM increases the survival rate of the flap

QUIZ 8
EXTENDED MATCHING QUESTIONS

For questions 8.41 to 8.45 please select the ONE MOST appropriate answer from list [A] to [K]. Each answer maybe used more than once or not at all.

The following is a list of cutaneous nerves of the lower limbs.

[A] Ilioinguinal nerve

[B] Anterior femoral cutaneous nerve

[C] Saphenous nerve

[D] Medial plantar nerve

[E] Calcaneal nerve

[F] Common peroneal nerve

[G] Lateral femoral cutaneous nerve

[H] Iliohypogastric nerve

[J] Posterior femoral cutaneous nerve

[K] Sural nerve

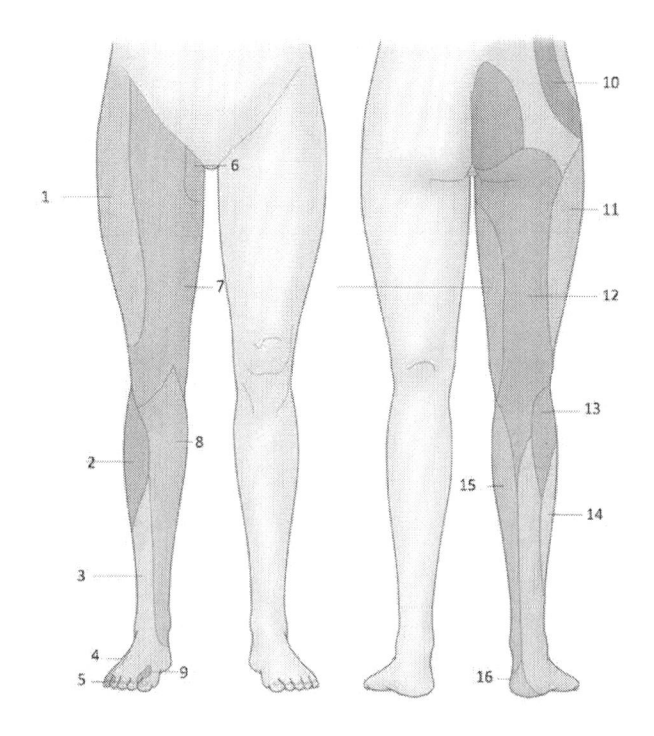

Please match the numbers on the on the diagram with the appropriate dermatome listed above.

Q 8.41
Dermatome 4

Q 8.42
Dermatome 8

Q 8.43
Dermatome 2

Q 8.44
Dermatome 1

Q 8.45
Dermatome 6

For questions 8.46 to 8.50 please select the ONE MOST appropriate answer from list [A] to [K]. Each answer maybe used more than once or not at all.

The following is a list of structures of the head.

[A] Temporalis muscle

[B] Ethmoid bone

[C] Supraorbital nerve

[D] Mental nerve

[E] Supratrochlear nerve

[F] Infraorbital vein

[G] Condylar process

[H] Vomer

[J] External auditory meatus

[K] Greater wing of sphenoid bone

Which one of the above corresponds to the ANNOTATION ON THE DIAGRAM below?

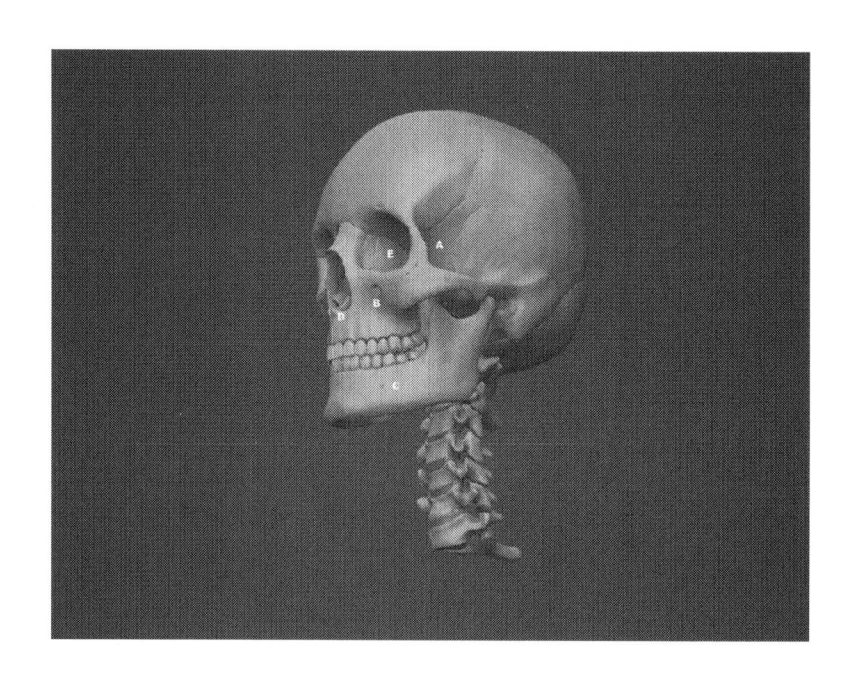

Q 8.46
Structure A?

Q 8.47
Which structure emerges from foramen C?

Q 8.48
Structure E?

Q 8.49
Which structure emerges from foramen B?

Q 8.50
What is the name of structure D?

QUIZ 8
ANSWERS

8.1
Answer D
Sixty percent of haemangiomas are expected to spontaneously resolve by 6 years of age; 705 at 7 years; 80% at 8 years and 90% at 9 years of age.

8.2
Answer B
The inferior oblique muscle separates the medial and nasal fat pads of the lower eyelid.

8.3
Answer B
The inferior oblique muscle is innervated by the inferior division of the oculomotor nerve.

8.4
Answer B
This is a classical description of the Kasabach-Merritt syndrome due to a haemangioendothelioma. The description given is of thrombocytopenia with disseminated intravascular coagulation (DIC).

8.5
Answer A
The normal inter-orbital distance is 23 – 28mm.

8.6
Answer C
The fascial compartments of the leg are the anterior, peroneal and superficial and deep posterior compartments. Despite the presence of the anterior wound, all four compartments need to be formally decompressed.

8.7
Answer C
Subcutaneous mastectomy involves excision of most of the breast tissue preserving the nipple-areolar complex and overlying skin. Skin-sparing mastectomy, on the other hand, involves excision of the breast and nipple-areolar complex and preserving the overlying skin flaps.

8.8
Answer B
DIEP flaps are associated with a higher rate of fat necrosis than free TRAM flaps. However, it is associated with less donor site morbidity as the functionof the rectus abdominis muscle is preserved.

8.9
Answer C
Simon's classification of gynaecomastia:
Grade 1: Mild increase in breast volume; no skin excess
Grade 2A: Moderate increase in volume; no excess skin
Grade 2B: Moderate increase in volume; skin excess; Grade 1 ptosis
Grade 3: Severe increase in volume; skin excess; Grade 2 or 3 ptosis

8.10
Answer B
The external auditory canal is a derivative of the first branchial cleft.

8.11
Answer A
Acetylcholine receptors are classified as nicotinic and muscarinic cholinergic receptors

8.12
Answer D
The facial nerve usually enter the muscles of facial expression on their deep surface except the mentalis, buccinator and the levator anguli superioris where it enters on the superficial surface

8.13
Answer D
Müller's muscle is a smooth muscle with sympathetic innervations.

8.14
Answer A
Basal cell carcinomas are by far the most common malignancy affecting the lower eyelid.

8.15
Answer C
The normal chondromastoid angle in an average adult is about 31.1° based on work by Da Silva Freitas et al.

8.16
Answer A
Smoking is not an absolute contraindication to microsurgery. It is not associated with greater flap loss but is associated with a higher rate of wound healing complications. Smoking after digital replantation is associated with a higher rate of failure.

8.17
Answer B
Dextran 40 is a low molecular weight polysaccharide. Its use in microsurgery is controversial since it can increase the rate of complication without increase patency rates. Its exact mechanism of action is unknown but it results in volume expansion and inhibits von Willebrand's factor. It can cause an anaphylaxis reaction.

8.18
Answer A
This classification is based on histological analysis.

8.19
Answer C
A tumour extending to the junction of the papillary and reticular dermis corresponds to Clark's level 3. It is not possible to determine the Breslow thickness from the information provided in the stem of the question. In an non-ulcerated lesion the Breslow thickness of the tumour is measured from the granular layer to the maximum depth of the tumour.

8.20
Answer C
Sentinel lymph node biopsy (SLNB) is useful in the detection of micrometases and hence in the staging of the disease. Although it does not improve the overall prognosis of the disease it has been shown to confer a survival benefit in patients with intermediate-thickness melanomas.

8.21
Answer D
By far, BCC's occur most commonly on the head and neck regions. Twenty-six percent of all BCC's occur on the nose.

8.22
Answer B
Isolated cleft palate occurs in 30% of patients with cleft lip and/or palate. The most common deformity is cleft lip with cleft palate (45%).

8.23
Answer C
The primary problem that intiates the Pierre-Robin sequence is a small jaw.

8.24
Answer C
Bone grafts placed in a heterotopic position (the recipient site is not normally occupied by bone) are more prone to failure.

8.25
Answer D
Alloderm is cadaveric human dermis processed to remove all the cellular elements leaving the collagen framework. Because the cellular elements are removed it is only minimally allergenic. It is useful as a temporary skin substitute.

8.26
Answer B
In' true' plagiocephaly the skull is shaped like a rhomboid (or parallelogram) whereas in 'positional' plagiocephaly the skull is shaped like a triangle with its apex lying on the affected side.

8.27
Answer A
Treacher Collins syndrome is an autosomal dominant bilateral confluent Tessier clefts 6 – 8.

8.28
Answer C
This is most likely hemifacial micromia since it is congenital and unilateral.

8.29
Answer D
Rectangular shaped expanders produce the greatest gain in expanded tissue area.

8.30
Answer C
Melanin is the chromophore used in hair removal.

8.31
Answer B
Intralesional steroids inhibit fibroblast proliferation and collagen production; stimulates collagenase activity.

8.32
Answer D

8.33
Answer D
Each osteon comprises of osteocytes and a central haversian canal that contains a nutrient vessel. Osteons are connected to each other by tranverse nutrient canals knowm as Volkmann's canals.

8.34
Answer C

8.35
Answer A
Patients with cutis laxa present with features of premature aging due to loose, inelastic skin. They don't have wound healing problems.

8.36
Answer D
Vacuum therapy decreases the concentration of metalloproteinases in the wound encouraging healing.

8.37
Answer A
Reverse-cutting needles have a flat surface on the inner side of the curve of the needle as opposed to conventional cutting needles that a sharp edge on the inner side of the curve of the needle.

8.38
Answer B
The most common site of metastasis of a tumour of the anterior two-thirds of the tongue is a level II lymph node although levels I and III are also at risk.

8.39
Answer A
The facial nerve is found 1cm deep and 1cm inferior to the tragal pointer.

8.40
Answer A
The deep inferior epigastric vessels are the dominant vessels of the TRAM flap. It is a Type II myocutaneous flap based on the Mathes and Nahai classification of muscle flaps and it is regarded as a type of autologous breast reconstruction. A delay procedure involving ligation of the deep inferior epigastric vessels 2-3 weeks prior to a pedicle TRAM increases the survival rate of the flap.

8.41
Answer K

8.42
Answer C

8.43
Answer F

8.44
Answer G

8.45
Answer A

8.46
Answer K

8.47
Answer D

8.48
Answer B

8.49
Answer F

8.50
Answer H

QUIZ 9
MULTIPLE CHOICE QUESTIONS

For questions 9.1 to 9.40 please the ONE most appropriate answer.

Q 9.1
Which structure does the orbital septum arise from?

[A] Levator aponeurosis

[B] Muller's muscles

[C] Orbital periosteum

[D] Orbicularis oculi

Q 9.2
Which one of the following muscles is innervated by the trochlear nerve?

[A] Medial rectus muscle

[B] Lateral rectus muscle

[C] Superior oblique muscle

[D] Inferior oblique muscle

Q 9.3
Which one of the following is NOT a muscle of the glabella region which produces the glabella furrows?

[A] Preseptal orbicularis oculi

[B] Procerus

[C] Depressor supercilii

[D] Corrugator supercilii

Q 9.4
When undergoing blepharoplasty, patients should be advised to stop all the following drugs EXCEPT?

[A] Nitrofurantoin

[B] Aspirin

[C] Vitamin E

[D] Garlic supplements

Q 9.5
Which ONE of the following is NOT a true retaining ligament of the face?

[A] Zygomatic ligament

[B] Masseteric ligament

[C] Lateral orbital thickening

[D] Mandibular retaining ligament

Q 9.6
How many fat compartments are there in the upper eyelids?

[A] 1

[B] 2

[C] 3

[D] 4

Q 9.7
Which of the following structures is the primary upper lid retractor?

[A] Muller's muscles

[B] Levator muscle

[C] Orbicularis oculi

[D] Orbital septum

Q 9.8
Which of the following is characteristic of the endothelium of a haemangioma?

[A] The endothelial cells are narrow and have a 'picket-fence' pattern of arrangement

[B] There is an increase in number of macrophages between the endothelial cells

[C] The endothelial cells have a longer lifespan than the normal

[D] There is an increase in the number of mast cells

Q 9.9
Which of the following is NOT a feature of Poland's syndrome?

[A] Loss of axillary hair

[B] It is only associated with defects of the soft tissues

[C] Can present with a sternal deformity on the contralateral side

[D] Syndactyly

Q 9.10
A 20 year-old patient presents with an open fracture of the left tibia with a 10cm gaping wound on the anterior aspect of the left leg. He is taken to theatre within 6 hours and the wound is adequately debrided left open and also undergoes internal fixation of the fractured tibia. Five hours post-operatively he complains of severe pain in the limb. A diagnosis of compartment syndrome is arrived at and he taken to theatre for fasciotomy. How many compartments need to be decompressed in this patient?

[A] 2

[B] 3

[C] 4

[D] 5

Q 9.11
A 54 year-old professional rock climber presents to the outpatient clinic after referral by a breast surgeon. She is due to undergo a right mastectomy for breast cancer and would like to have an immediate breast reconstruction. She is likely to require adjuvant radiotherapy following the procedure. On examination, she has an intact and well developed latissimus dorsi on the right side, the anterior edge of which is palpable. She also has a redundant tissue on the lower abdomen and there are no abdominal scars. Which of the following do you think is the most appropriate methods of reconstruction for this patient?

[A] A breast implant reconstruction

[B] A breast expander reconstruction followed by exchange for a definitive implant after expansion

[C] A pedicled latissimus dorsi muscle and implant reconstruction

[D] A DIEP flap reconstruction

Q 9.12
Which of the following drugs is NOT regarded as a cause of gynaecomastia?

[A] Amoxicillin

[B] Metronidazole

[C] Enalapril

[D] Marijuana

Q 9.13
A 67 year-old gentleman present with a large basal cell carcinoma on his left temple. On surgical excision the temporal branch of the facial nerve is identified and preserved. Which plane is the temporal branch of the facial nerve found in this region of the face?

[A] Within the subcutaneous tissue

[B] Deep to the superficial temporoparietal fascia

[C] Deep to the deep temporal fascia

[D] Deep to the temporal muscle

Q 9.14
Which of the following is NOT a component of the posterior lamella of the upper eyelid?

[A] Conjunctiva

[B] Levator aponeurosis

[C] Pretarsal fibres of the orbicularis oculi

[D] Tarsus

Q 9.15
Which ONE of the following nerves is not anatomically related to the submandibular gland?

[A] Marginal mandibular nerve

[B] Hypoglossal nerve

[C] Spinal accessory nerve

[D] Lingual nerve

Q 9.16
Which of the following statements is FALSE?

[A] Glottic malignancies have a greater risk of metastases than supraglottic malignancies

[B] Elective selective neck dissection is usually recommended for Stage I and II tongue cancers

[C] Extracapsular extension of cervical nodal metastasis is an indication for postoperative radiotherapy

[D] Bilateral jugular vein invasion by confirmed cervical metastastic nodal disease of a squamous cell carcinoma of the right pinna is a relative contraindication to surgery

Q 9.17
At what age would you consider performing a total ear reconstruction for a newborn with severe unilateral microtia?

[A] In the first weeks of life

[B] At 1 year of age

[C] At 6 years of age

[D] At 12 years of age

Q 9.18
Which of the following is NOT true regarding a reperfusion injury?

[A] Occurs secondary to the accumulation of free radicals in the devascularised tissue

[B] The reperfusion injury classically occurs prior to the re-establishment of perfusion

[C] Results in endothelial cell swelling and damage

[D] More likely to occur in tissues with muscle

Q 9.19

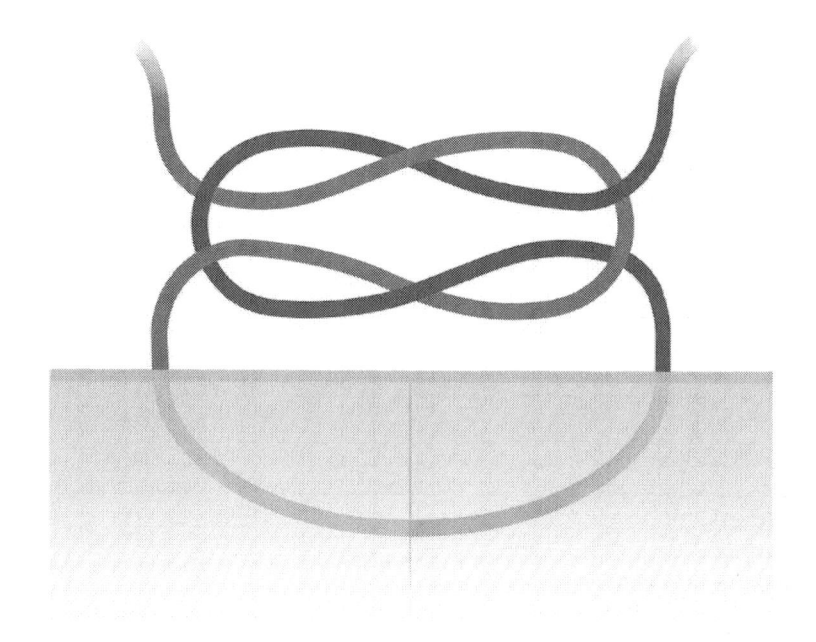

Which type of surgical knot is illustrated above?

[A] Surgeon's knot

[B] Granny knot

[C] Reef Knot

[D] Sliding knot

Q 9.20
A 56 year gentleman is referred to your Clinic with a biopsy-proven SCC on the right pinna which is adherent to the underlying cartilage. The lesion has a diameter of 15mm. The of the following is the BEST surgical option for treating this patient is?

[A] Excision of the lesion with a 4mm margin and preserving the perichondrium overlying the cartilage

[B] Excision of the lesion with a 4mm margin and excising the underlying cartilage and reconstructing the defect with a full thickness skin graft

[C] Excision of the lesion with a 6mm margin and preserving the perichondrium overlying the cartilage

[D] Excision of the lesion with an 8mm margin and excising the underlying cartilage

Q 9.21
A 57 year gentleman has had a 2.1cm well-differentiated SCC excised from the left lower leg? What is the likely overall risk of this patient developing metastasis?

[A] 9%

[B] 15%

[C] 23%

[D] 30%

Q 9.22
What is the blood supply to the hard palate?

[A] Lesser palatine artery

[B] Greater palatine artery

[C] Ascending pharyngeal artery

[D] Ascending palatine branch of the facial artery

Q 9.23
A 16 year-old female patient presents to the outpatient department with a history of 2cm in diameter well-circumscribed round defect on the upper right side of the forehead which she has had from birth. On examination, it appears to be a defect underlying the skin. The base of the defect feels bony. The frontalis muscle appears to be normal surrounding the defect but is distinctly absent within the defect. Which of the following is a MOST likely diagnosis?

[A] Hemifacial microsomia

[B] Hemifacial atrophy

[C] Cutis aplasia congenita

[D] Acquired defect secondary to birth trauma

Q 9.24
With regards to tissue expansion which one of the following statements is FALSE?

[A] A defect of up to 50% of the scalp can be reconstructed with tissue expansion

[B] The area of tissue available following tissue expansion is calculated by subtracting the base diameter of the expander from the circumference

[C] Should never be used in the lower limbs

[D] Multiple tissue expanders can be used simultaneously

Q 9.25
Which of the following is NOT a property of the 'ideal' dressing?

[A] Protection of the wound from physical harm

[B] Decrease the formation of granulation tissue which may impair wound healing

[C] Promote epithelialization

[D] Have antibacterial properties

Q 9.26
What is the peak tensile strength expected for healed wound?

[A] 50%

[B] 60%

[C] 80%

[D] 95%

Q 9.27
A 57 year-old gentleman has just undergone wide excision of a 3mm Breslow thickness melanoma from his back along with a positive sentinel node biopsy from his left axilla but no palpable lymphadenopathy. A subsequent staging CT scan reported no distant metastases. Based on the AJCC classification, what is the stage of his disease?

[A] Stage 2A

[B] Stage 2C

[C] Stage 3A

[D] Stage 3B

Q 9.28
Which ONE of the following is NOT a useful modality to treat basal cell carcinomas?

[A] Photodynamic therapy

[B] Shave excision

[C] Cryotherapy

[D] Radiotherapy

Q 9.29
Which ONE of the following is contraindicated in the treatment of a BCC on the back of a patient with Gorlin's syndrome?

[A] Excision biopsy

[B] Topical 5-Fluorouracil

[C] Photodynamic therapy

[D] Radiotherapy

Q 9.30
Gorlin's syndrome arises from a defect in which ONE of the following genes?

[A] BRAF

[B] VEGF

[C] VEGF-C

[D] PTCH-1

Q 9.31
A mutation in which ONE of the following genes increases the likelihood of a response with vemurafenib (a targeted therapy agent) in patients with Stage IV melanoma?

[A] VEGF-C

[B] BRAF

[C] PTCH-1

[D] BRCA-2

Q 9.32
Which ONE of the following category of drugs used in the treatment of Stage IV melanoma does the drug, ipilimumab, belong to?

[A] Chemotherapy

[B] Targeted therapy

[C] Immunotherapy

[D] Antimicrobial therapy

Q 9.33
A 63-year patient with Stage III melanoma presents with an in-transit metastasis adjacent to scar of the primary tumour. What is the most appropriate course of action to treat this patient?

[A] Re-stage the patient with a CT scan prior to embarking on further treatment

[B] Proceed immediately to excision of the subcutaneous metastasis

[C] Refer her to a medical oncologist for chemotherapy

[D] Refer her to a clinical oncologist for radiotherapy

Q 9.34
Which ONE of the following is an example of an immunotherapy drug used in the treatment of Stage IV melanoma?

[A] Vemurafenib

[B] Dabrafenib

[C] Ipilimumab

[D] Dacarbazine

Q 9.35
Which ONE of the following is NOT a recognised modality for surgically treating lymphoedema?

[A] Liposuction

[B] Free vascularized lymph node transfers

[C] Lympho-venous anastomoses

[D] Lymphatic vessel grafts

Q 9.36
How would you classify a patient with total paralysis of the left side of the face using the House-Brackmann scale?

[A] Grade III

[B] Grade V

[C] Grade VI

[D] Grade VII

Q 9.37
All of the following steps are indicated in the management of extravasation injuries EXCEPT?

[A] Stop the transfusion

[B] Flush the line/device

[C] Aspirate as much of the residual drugs as possible

[D] Mark and measure the extravasated area

Q 9.38
Which of the following structures denotes the upper border of a level III neck dissection?

[A] The posterior belly of digastric muscle

[B] The omohyoid muscle

[C] Base of the skull

[D] The bifurcation of the carotid artery

Q 9.39
With regards to the treatment of bilateral cleft lip which of the following statements is CORRECT?

[A] Presurgical orthopaedic appliances are always used

[B] The prolabium is the skeletal remnant of the medial nasal processes of the frontonasal process

[C] The Millard technique of cleft lip repair cannot be used since it is useful in unilateral cleft lip repair

[D] The Manchester repair is used when the prolabium is relatively small

Q 9.40

A free vascularised fibula used to reconstruct a tibial defect mainly heals by which one of the following processes?

[A] Osseoconduction

[B] Incorporation

[C] Oseoinduction

[D] Osteogenesis

QUIZ 9
EXTENDED MATCHING QUESTIONS

For questions 9.41 to 9.45 please select the ONE MOST appropriate answer from list [A] to [K]. Each answer maybe used more than once or not at all.

The following is a list of embryological structures of the head and neck.

[A] First branchial arch
[B] Second branchial arch
[C] Third branchial arch
[D] Fourth branchial arch
[E] Fifth branchial arch
[F] First pharyngeal groove
[G] Second branchial groove
[H] First pharyngeal pouch
[J] Second branchial pouch
[K] Third branchial pouch

Please select the best answer from the list above.

Q 9.41
The external auditory meatus is derived from?

Q 9.42
The trigeminal nerve is derived from?

Q 9.43
The Eustachian tube is derived from?

Q 9.44
The facial nerve is derived from?

Q 9.45
The maxilla is derived from?

For questions 9.46 to 9.50 please select the ONE MOST appropriate answer from list [A] to [K]. Each answer maybe used more than once or not at all.

The following is a list of local flaps.

[A] Triple-Rhomboid flaps
[B] Bilobed flap
[C] H-flaps
[D] Bipedicled advancement flap
[E] Simple advancement flap
[F] V-Y advancement flap
[G] Multiple y-V flaps
[H] Simple transposition flap
[J] Rotation flap
[K] V-T flap

Which one of the following flaps outlined above is best for the reconstruction of the each of the defects outlined below.

Q 9.46
A lesion of the middle third of the right nasal sidewall?

Q 9.47
A 2 cm defect of the centre of the forehead?

Q 9.48
A 1 cm in diameter defect of the left side of the nasal tip?

Q 9.49
A 3.5 cm defect of the medial proximal third of the leg?

Q 9.50
A 9 cm in diameter circular defect in the centre of the back?

QUIZ 9
ANSWERS

9.1
Answer C
The orbital septum is a firm, fibrous structure which is deep to the orbicularis muscle and arises from the orbital rim periosteum.

9.2
Answer C
The superior oblique muscle is the only extraocular muscle innervated by the trochlear nerve (the fourth cranial nerve).

9.3
Answer A
The muscles of the glabella region are:
 1. Procerus
 2. Depressor supercilii
 3. Corrugator supercilii

9.4
Answer A
Nitrofurantoin is an antibiotic and does not predispose to bleeding. Aspirin, Vitamin /e and Garlic supplements can predispose patients to bleed excessively which may result in haematoma or extensive bruising.

9.5
Answer B
True retaining ligaments are easily identifiable and connect the dermis to the underlying periosteum. The zygomatic ligament, lateral orbital thickening and the mandibular ligaments are true retaining ligaments. False retaining ligaments are more diffuse and connect the superficial and deep facial fascia. The masseteric ligament is a false retaining ligament of the cheek.

9.6
Answer B
There are 2 fat compartments in the upper eyelid.

9.7
Answer B
The levator muscle is the primary retractor of the upper lid.

9.8
Answer D
Histologically, haemangiomas consist of plump, hyperplastic endothelial cells which have a rapid turnover rate. There is an increase in the number of mast cells.

9.9
Answer B
Poland's syndrome can affect the soft tissues and well as the underlying skeleton. It may present with a deformity of the contralateral sternum due to rotation of the sternum.

9.10
Answer C
The fascial compartments of the leg are the anterior, peroneal and superficial and deep posterior compartments. Despite the presence of the anterior wound, all four compartments need to be formally decompressed.

9.11
Answer D
An expander/implant reconstruction is not ideal for the reconstruction of this patient's breast since it is likely she that she would need radiotherapy. Since she is a professional rock climber, a latissimus dorsi mucle and implant reconstruction is not ideal either.

9.12
Answer A
Metronidazole, enalapril and marijuana are all known to cause gynaecomastia.

9.13
Answer B
The temporal branch of the facial nerve lies along Pitanguy's line running from 1cm inferior to the inter-tragal point to a point 1cm above the lateral eyebrow. Lateral to the lateral canthus of the eye it is found deep to the superficial temporal fascia but superficial to the deep temporal fascia.

9.14
Answer C
The orbicularis oculi is a component of the anterior lamella. Components of the posterior lamella are the conjunctiva, levator aponeurosis, Müller's muscle and the tarsus.

9.15
Answer C
The spinal accessory nerve is not closely related to the submandibular gland.

9.16
Answer A
Supraglottic malignancies have a higher metastatic rate than glottis malignancies. Elective selective neck dissection is usually recommended for Stage I and II tongue cancers because of a high risk of metastasis. Extracapsular extension of cervical nodal metastasis is an indication for postoperative radiotherapy

9.17
Answer C
The rib cartilages used in total ear reconstruction are only large enough in children 6 years of age to create an adult size ear.

9.18
Answer B
Reperfusion injury occurs after re-establishment of perfusion to the tissue. Muscles are more intolerant to ischaemia than skin. It occurs due to the accumulation of free radicals in the devascularised tissue resulting in endothelial swelling and damage.

9.19
Answer B
The grsnny knot is an unstable knot by configuration.

9.20
Answer D
Although the size of the lesion in case is less than 2cm it is present in a high risk area making it a high risk SCC. This should be excised with at least a 6mm margin. Since the tumour was attached to the underlying cartilage, this should be also be excised with the specimen to ensure adequate tumour clearance.

9.21
Answer A
The risk of a patient with a well-differentiated T2 lesion developing metastases is 7-9%.

9.22
Answer B
The greater palatine artery which is a branch of the maxillary artery is supplies the hard palate.

9.23
Answer D
Of the options given, the most likely diagnosis is a soft tissue defect secondary to birth trauma. Cutis aplasia congenita, by definition, involves a congenital defect of the overlying skin. This defect, as described, is too localised and well demarcated to be either hemifacial microsomia or hemifacial atrophy.

9.24
Answer C
Tissue expanders are used in the lower limbs, however, there is a higher rate of complications such as extrusion compared to expanders used on the upper limb.

9.25
Answer B
The formation of granulation tissue is essential for secondary wound healing. Over-granulation is problematic and needs treatment.

9.26
Answer C
The peak tensile strength of a healed wound is about 80% of the pre-injury level.

9.27
Answer C
This patient presents with an intermediate-thickness melanoma with micrometastases. In view of this, this is best staged as Stage 3A.

9.28
Answer B
Shave excision is likely to incompletely excise the BCC hence it is not a suitable modality for treatment. Excision however, is the ideal modality of treatment.

9.29
Answer D
Radiotherapy is contraindicated for the treatment of BCCs in patients with Gorlin's syndrome as it can stimulate the development of more BCCs.

9.30
Answer D

9.31
Answer B
Patients with melanomas with the BRAF mutation are more likely to respond to the targeted therapy drugs like vemurafenib.

9.32
Answer C
Ipilimumab belongs to the immunotherapy class of drugs.

9.33
Answer A
This patient needs to be re-staged to rule out distant metastases prior to surgical treatment. This patient should also be referred to a medical oncologist but there is no role for chemotherapy in this case.

9.34
Answer C
Dacarbazine is a chemotherapeutic drug whereas vemurafenib and dabrafenib are targeted agents.

9.35
Answer D

9.36
Answer C
The House-Brackmann scale for the classification of facial palsy is from Grade I to Grade VI. Total paralysis falls into Grade VI.

9.37
Answer B
With extravasation injuries, under no circumstances should the line/device be flushed as this may propagate the agent deeper or widespread into the tissues.

9.38
Answer D
The superior border of level III is the bifurcation of the carotid artery, the inferior border is the omohyoid muscle, the anterior border is the posterior edge of the sternohyoid muscle and the posterior border is the posterior edge of the sternocleidomastoid muscle.

9.39
Answer D
In bilateral cleft lip the prolabium is the soft tissue remnant of the medial nasal processes of the frontonasal process. The skeletal element is the premaxilla. If the prolabium is relatively large, the Millard repair can be used. If the prolabium is relatively small the Manchester repair is used.

9.40
Answer D
This is the predominant process whereby vascularised bone grafts heal by the formation of new bone by the osteocytes within the graft itself.

9.41
Answer F

9.42
Answer A

9.43
Answer H

9.44
Answer B

9.45
Answer A

9.46
Answer E

9.47
Answer C

9.48
Answer B

9.49
Answer D

9.50
Answer A

QUIZ 10
MULTIPLE CHOICE QUESTIONS

For questions 10.1 to 10.40 please the ONE most appropriate answer.

Q 10.1

The extended area of skin which is perfused by a named artery after a delaying procedure is known as the

[A] Anatomical territory of the artery

[B] Dynamic territory of the artery

[C] Potential territory of the artery

[D] Choke area of the artery

Q 10.2
A rigidly fixed fracture of the shaft of the 4th metacarpal bone heals by which of the following processes?

[A] Primary bone healing

[B] Secondary bone healing

[C] Intramembranous ossification

[D] Endochondral ossification

Q 10.3
Vacuum-assisted wound closure work using the following techniques EXCEPT?

[A] Increases the rate of granulation tissue formation

[B] Direct suction on the wound edges result in wound contraction

[C] Decreases the bacterial load of the wound

[D] Increases the concentration of tissue metalloproteinases in the wound

Q 10.4
A new Class IV Nd:YAG laser is available for use in your department. Which of the following statements is TRUE?

[A] Lasers are rated by their potential to induce ocular damage

[B] Lasers are rated by their depth of penetrance of solid lead shields

[C] The smoke fumes generated by the use of lasers are not as hazardous as that produced by electrocautery

[D] Flammable liquids can be safely used with lasers since the heat produced is deep within the tissues

Q 10.5
A tissue expander is being inserted under the scalp for the reconstruction of a skin grafted area of 7 x 7cm. Ideally, where should the incision be made for the insertion of the expander?

[A] Along the edge of the skin graft

[B] A W-shaped incision within the skin grafted area

[C] A radial incision outside of the skin grafted area

[D] An incision parallel to the edge of the skin a distance equal to one diameter away from the edge of the skin graft

Q 10.6
Which of the following is characteristic of Romberg's hemifacial atrophy?

[A] It presents after 5 years of age

[B] It has an autosomal pattern of inheritance

[C] It is associated with a positive family history

[D] The underlying bony skeleton is characteristically not affected

Q 10.7
A 65 year-old gentleman has a BCC incompletely excised from his left cheek. What is the likely chance that this patient would have a recurrence of the lesion within the next 5 years?

[A] 5%

[B] 15%

[C] 30%

[D] 60%

Q 10.8
A 70 year-old gentleman has a BCC incompletely excised from his left cheek. What is the likely chance that residual tumour would be identified in the tissue following re-excision using standard histological sectioning techniques?

[A] 15%

[B] 30%

[C] 50%

[D] 100%

Q 10.9
What is the normal chondromastoid angle in an average adult?

[A] 5°

[B] 106°

[C] 31°

[D] 47°

Q 10.10
An 80 year-old gentleman had a squamous cell carcinoma of the lower lip excised. The resultant defect involved about 25% of the lateral aspect of the lower lip and included the oral commissure of the mouth. Which of the following ids the BEST reconstructive option of this defect?

[A] Abbe flap

[B] Direct closure

[C] Eastlander flap

[D] Karapandzic flap

Q 10.11
Acetylcholine is the neurotransmitter which is present between the pre- and ganglionic fibres of the facial nerve. Acetylcholine is attaches to which of the following receptors?

[A] Nicotinic

[B] Dopaminergic

[C] GABAergic

[D] Histaminergic

Q 10.12
The external auditory canal is a derivative of the following embryological structures?

[A] The first branchial arch

[B] The fist branchial cleft

[C] The second branchial arch

[D] The second branchial cleft

Q 10.13
Which of the following drugs is NOT useful in the treatment of gynaecomastia?

[A] Tamoxifen

[B] Testosterone

[C] Danazole

[D] Progesterone

Q 10.14
A 26 year old male student presents to you with increased breast size. He says that he developed this since he was 14 years of age and it has not reduced in size since. On examination both breasts are symmetrical and moderately enlarged with noticeable skin excess and mild ptosis. What grade would this fall under in the Simon's classification of gynaecomastia?

[A] Grade 1

[B] Grade 2

[C] Grade 2B

[D] Grade 3

Q 10.15
What proportion of haemangiomas is expected to spontaneously resolve at 7 years of age?

[A] 40%

[B] 50%

[C] 60%

[D] 70%

Q 10.16
How many fat compartments are there in the lower eyelid?

[A] 1

[B] 2

[C] 3

[D] 4

Q 10.17
Where is the lacrimal gland situated?

[A] In the lateral compartment of the upper eyelid

[B] In the medial compartment of the upper eyelid

[C] In the medial compartment of the lower eyelid

[D] In the lateral compartment of the lower eyelid

Q 10.18
Which of the following structures is located between the middle and nasal fat pads of the upper eyelid?

[A] The trochlear of the inferior oblique muscle

[B] The medial rectus muscle

[C] The lateral rectus muscle

[D] The trochlear of the superior oblique muscle

Q 10.19
Which of the following is NOT a function of the superior oblique muscle in relation to eyeball movement?

[A] Oblique rotation

[B] Internal rotation

[C] Depression

[D] Lateral rotation

Q 10.20
Which ONE of the following category of drugs used in the treatment of Stage IV melanoma does the drug, ipilimumab, belong to?

[A] Chemotherapy

[B] Targeted therapy

[C] Immunotherapy

[D] Antimicrobial therapy

Q 10.21
Gorlin's syndrome arises from a defect in which ONE of the following genes?

[A] BRAF

[B] VEGF

[C] VEGF-C

[D] PTCH-1

Q 10.22
Which of the following flaps is NOT suitable for the coverage of defects around the knee?

[A] Pedicled soleus flap

[B] Medial gastocnenius muscle flap

[C] Lateral gastrocnemius muscle flap

[D] Saphenous fasciocutaneous flap

Q 10.23
Which of the following is NOT a characteristic feature of the nasal deformity associated with a cleft lip?

[A] A kink of the lateral crus of the lower alar cartilage on the contralateral side

[B] Separation of the domes of the alar cartilages at the tip of the nose

[C] Retrodisplacement of the nasal base on the ipsilateral side

[D] Deviation of the nasal spine away from the cleft side

Q 10.24
With regards to cleft lip and palate repair, which of the following statements is TRUE?

[A] The cleft lip component should be repaired in the first 48 hours after birth to prevent long term scarring and deformity

[B] The cleft palate component should be repaired in the first 48 hours to prevent disturbance of midfacial growth in the first year of life

[C] Presurgical orthopaedics is mandatory in the first 48 hours of life

[D] The Schweckendiek technique recommends hard palatal repair at approximately 8 years of age

Q 10.25
At what age would you consider performing a total ear reconstruction for a newborn with severe unilateral microtia?

[A] In the first weeks of life

[B] At 1 year of age

[C] At 6 years of age

[D] At 12 years of age

Q 10.26
Using the Regnault classification of breast ptosis which of the following MOST closely describes a third degree breast ptosis?

[A] The nipple lies at the level of the inframammary fold (IMF) but the major portion of the breast tissue lies below the IMF

[B] The nipple and the most dependent portion of the breast lies below the inframammary fold

[C] The nipple lies below the inframammary fold but above the most dependent portion of the breast

[D] The nipple lies above the inframammary fold

Q 10.27
The sounds of which of the following consonants are regarded as fricatives?

[A] S

[B] B

[C] P

[D] M

Q 10.28
Which of the following statements is FALSE regarding the role of TGF-β in normal wound healing?

[A] Attracts fibroblasts into the wound

[B] Stimulates collagen production by fibroblasts

[C] Stimulates angiogenesis

[D] Is produced by macrophages and does not play a role in the attraction of macrophages into the wound

Q 10.29
Which of the following statements most accurately describes the course of the spinal accessory nerve as it courses through the neck?
[A] It crosses the sternocleidomastoid muscle in the upper-middle third towards the middle-lower third of the trapezius

[B] It crosses the sternocleidomastoid muscle in the middle-lower third towards the middle-lower third of the trapezius

[C] It crosses the sternocleidomastoid muscle in the upper-middle third towards the upper-middle third of the trapezius

[D] It crosses the sternocleidomastoid muscle in the middle-lower third towards the upper-middle third of the trapezius

Q 10.30
What is the main functional muscle of the soft palate producing velopharyngeal closure?

[A] Tensor veli palatini

[B] Levator veli palatini

[C] Muscularis uvulae

[D] Stylopharyngeus

Q 10.31
All of the following are clinical features of true plagiocephaly EXCEPT?

[A] The skull is triangular shaped

[B] Prominence of the ipsilateral cheek

[C] The distance between the lateral orbit and the ear is decreased on the ipsilateral side

[D] Prominence of the contralateral brow

Q 10.32
Which ONE of the following can potentially penetrate deepest into the skin?

[A] UVA

[B] UVB

[C] UVC

[D] Infra-red light

Q 10.33
Which of the following is a characteristic feature of Mobius syndrome?

[A] Bilateral facial atrophy

[B] Bilateral involvement of the cranial nerves VII only

[C] Bilateral involvement of the cranial nerves VI and VII

[D] It is associated with mental underdevelopment

Q 10.34
Which of the following is NOT true of keratoacanthomas?

[A] They demonstrate rapid growth

[B] They can resolve spontaneously

[C] Can be easily differentiated from squamous cell carcinomas by histological examination

[D] They are associated with the Ferguson-Smith syndrome

Q 10.35
Cleft lip and palate deformities are surgically primarily repaired in the first year of life. This is done for the following reasons EXCEPT?

[A] For cosmesis

[B] To improve feeding and nutrition

[C] To prevent subsequent impairment in mid-facial growth and development

[D] To prevent abnormal speech

Q 10.36
The wavelength of ultraviolet light in terrestrial sunlight is most likely to be?

[A] 290-400nm

[B] 400-700nm

[C] 700-850nm

[D] More than 900nm

Q 10.37
Which of the following structures can be found to have the most yellow colour intra-operatively during upper lid blepharoplasty?

[A] The lacrimal gland

[B] The medial fat pad

[C] The middle fat pad

[D] The levator aponeurosis

Q 10.38
Which of the following is an accurate description of a Grade IIIc lower limb injury based on the Gustilo and Anderson classification?

[A] A high energy injury with extensive soft tissue damage

[B] A high energy injury with extensive soft tissue damage with periosteal stripping and bone exposure

[C] A high energy injury with extensive soft tissue damage, bony exposure and division of the tibial vessels

[D] A high energy injury with extensive soft tissue damage, bony exposure requiring soft tissue coverage with injury to the tibial nerve

Q 10.39
A primary SCC occurring in which of the following sites has the WORST prognosis (assuming that all other factors are constant)?

[A] Lower leg

[B] Penis

[C] Lower lip

[D] A chronic ulcer

Q 10.40
Which of the following statements regarding Warthin's tumour is FALSE?

[A] Common found in the tail of the parotid gland

[B] 10% are bilateral

[C] Is a malignant tumour of the parotid gland

[D] Treated by superficial parotidectomy

QUIZ 10
EXTENDED MATCHING QUESTIONS

For questions 10.41 to 10.45 please select the ONE MOST appropriate answer from list [A] to [K]. Each answer maybe used more than once or not at all.

The following are anatomical zones of the hand.

[A] Zone I
[B] Zone II
[C] Zone III
[D] Zone IV
[E] Zone V
[F] Zone VI
[G] Zone VII
[H] Zone VIII
[J] Zone IX
[K] Zone X

Q 10.41
Which of the above is also known as the zone of 'no man's land' on the flexor aspect of the hand?

Q 10.42
Which flexor zone corresponds to the anatomical level of the carpus?

Q 10.43
The level of the A1 pulley corresponds to the proximal line of which flexor zone?

Q 10.44
Which extensor zone corresponds to the level of the extensor retinaculum?

Q 10.45
Which extensor zone corresponds to the level of the metacarpophalangeal joints?

For questions 10.46 to 10.50 please select the ONE MOST appropriate answer from list [A] to [K]. Each answer maybe used more than once or not at all.

The following is a list of pioneers in flap surgery.

[A] Bakamjian
[B] Buncke
[C] Daniel/Taylor
[D] Tansini
[E] Holmstrom
[F] Song
[G] Soutar
[H] Koshima
[J] Townsend
[K] McGregor

Which of the above pioneers in flap surgery is/are credited with the following flaps? Please select only one answer from the list above.

Q 10.46
Pedicled latissimus dorsi flap?

Q 10.47
Deltopectoral flap?

Q 10.48
Lateral arm flap?

Q 10.49
Pedicled transverse rectus abdominis flap for breast reconstruction?

Q 10.50 Anterolateral flap?

QUIZ 10
ANSWERS

10.1
Answer C
The potential territory of a named artery is the extended area of skin that is supplied by the artery after undergoing a delaying procedure.

10.2
Answer A
This fracture would heal by the process of primary bone healing without callus formation. Intramembranous ossification is a process of bone formation by the deposition of bone within a vascularised, membranous template.

10.3
Answer D
Vacuum therapy decreases the concentration of metalloproteinases in the wound encouraging healing.

10.4
Answer A
Lasers are rated by their potential to induce ocular damage. Because the smoke fumes may contain traces of blood and potentially viruses, special laser quality masks must be worn. Flammable prep must not be used.

10.5
Answer B

Ideally the incision should be within the skin graft since this is expected to be excised anyway. An incision along the margin of the skin graft may have an increased risk of implant extrusion. Any incision away from the skin graft within the normal tissue may compromise the perfusion of the expander skin flap.

10.6
Answer A
Romberg's hemifacial atrophy usually presents after 5 years of age (usually in the early teen years). It is progressive and the disease usually 'burns out' in the mid-twenties. It is not associated with a positive family history and occurs sporadically. It is thought to be due to a viral infection or an abnormality of the sympathetic nervous system. It presents with progreesive, localised atrophy of the soft tissues of the face and may involve the underlying skeleton. It may present with a sharp depression of the forehead known as the 'coup de sabre'.

10.7
Answer C
The likely chance of a recurrence of the tumour following an incompletely excised BCC over the subsequent 2- 5 years is 30 – 40%.

10.8
Answer C
Re-excision of incompletely excised BCC's revealed the presence of residual tumour in 45 – 54% of cases using standard histological sectioning techniques.

10.9
Answer C
The normal chondromastoid angle in an average adult is about 31.1° based on work by Da Silva Freitas et al.

10.10
Answer C
The Eastlander is similar to the Abbe flap but it is performed in one stage and suitable for reconstructing defects of the lateral upper or lower lips that involve the oral commissure.

10.11
Answer A
Acetylcholine receptors are classified as nicotinic and muscarinic cholinergic receptors

10.12
Answer B
The external auditory canal is a derivative of the first branchial cleft.

10.13
Answer D
Tamxofen can reduce gynaecomastia in middle-aged men, testosterone can be used to treat gynaecomastia in patients with testicular failure. Danazol can reduce the pain associated with gynaecomastia and also reduce reduce the extent of gynaecomastia.

10.14
Answer C
Simon's classification of gynaecomastia:
Grade 1: Mild increase in breast volume; no skin excess
Grade 2A: Moderate increase in volume; no excess skin
Grade 2B: Moderate increase in volume; skin excess; Grade 1 ptosis
Grade 3: Severe increase in volume; skin excess; Grade 2 or 3 ptosis

10.15
Answer D
Sixty percent of haemangiomas are expected to spontaneously resolve by 6 years of age; 705 at 7 years; 80% at 8 years and 90% at 9 years of age.

10.16
Answer C
There are 3 fat compartments in the lower eyelid.

10.17
Answer A
The lacrimal gland is located in the lateral compartment of the upper eyelid. It maybe mistaken for a third fat pocket and inadvertently damaged. The upper eyelid had only 2 fat compartments as opposed to the lower eyelid which has 3.

10.18
Answer D
The trochlear of the superior oblique muscle lies between the middle and nasal fat pads of the upper eyelid. It maybe damaged during blepharoplasty.

10.19
Answer A
The primary action of the superior oblique muscle is internal rotation of the eyeball. The secondary action is depression and the tertiary action is lateral rotation.

10.20
Answer C
Ipilimumab belongs to the immunotherapy class of drugs.

10.21
Answer D

10.22
Answer A
The soleus muscle flap is appropriate for the coverage of defects of the middle third of the leg. The medial or lateral heads of the gastrocnemius muscle maybe used depending on the location and extent of the defect. In general, the medial head of the gastrocnemius muscle is used more frequently since it tends to be slightly longer than the lateral head.

10.23
Answer A
The features of the nasal deformity associates with a cleft lip are:
- Deviation of the nasal spine away from the cleft side
- A kink of the lateral crus of the lower alar cartilage on the *cleft* side
- Separation of the domes of the alar cartilages at the tip of the nose
- Retrodisplacement of the nasal base on the ipsilateral side
- Dislocation of the upper lateral cartilage from the lower lateral cartilage on the cleft side
- Flattening and displacement of the nasal bone on the cleft side

10.24
Answer D
With the Schweckendiek technique the lip and soft palate are repaired before 1 year of age and hard palate is repaired at about 8 years of age.

10.25
Answer C
The rib cartilages used in total ear reconstruction are only large enough in children 6 years of age to create an adult size ear.

10.26
Answer B
Regnault classification of breast ptosis:
First degree ptosis: The nipple lies above the inframammary fold
Second degree ptosis: The nipple lies below the inframammary fold but above the most dependent portion of the breast
Third degree ptosis: The nipple and the most dependent portion of the breast lies below the inframammary fold
Pseudo-ptosis: The nipple lies at the level of the inframammary fold (IMF) but the major portion of the breast tissue lies below the IMF.

10.27
Answer A
The consonants F and S are fricatives whereas B and P are plosives. M and N are nasal consonants.

10.28
Answer D
TGF-β is a growth factor which attracts both fibroblasts and macrophages. It stimulates the production of extracellar matrix by fibroblasts and induces angiogenesis.

10.29
Answer A
The spinal accessory nerve crosses the sternocleidomastoid muscle in the upper-middle third towards the middle-lower third of the trapezius 5cm above the clavicle. It is particularly prone to damage in cervical block dissections.

10.30
Answer B
The levator veli palatini originates from around the Eustachian tube and inserts into the palatine aponeurosis of the soft palate. As its name suggests, it elevates the soft palate and is very important in achieving velopharyngeal closure.

10.31
Answer B
In' true' plagiocephaly the skull is shaped like a rhomboid (or parallelogram) whereas in 'positional' plagiocephaly the skull is shaped like a triangle with its apex lying on the affected side.

10.32
Answer C
The depth of penetration of light into the skin depends on the wavelength. The shorter the wavelength, the deep it penetrates. UVC has the shortest wavelength (200-290nm)of the options provided.

10.33
Answer C
Mobius syndrome is a rare congenital neurological disorder characterised by the underdevelopment of cranial nerves VI and VII bilaterally. These patients characteristically have normal intelligence but an expressionless face.

10.34
Answer C
Keratoacanthomas demonstrate rapid growth and are known to resolve spontaneously. Ferguson-Smith syndrome is an autosomal dominant condition that presents with multiple self-healing epitheliomas. Keratoacanthomas are difficult to differentiate from squamous cell carcinomas clinically and even histologically.

10.35
Answer C
Cleft lip and palate procedures are undertaken for the following reasons:
- To look good
- To feed well
- For good speech
- To hear well (insertion of grommets in selected cases)
- For good dentition
- So that the patient can integrate well socially

10.36
Answer A
Terrestrial sunlight contains UV radiation of wavelengths between 290 and 400nm.

10.37
Answer C
The medial fat pad is pale in colour compared to the middle fat pad in the upper eyelid.

10.38
Answer C
A Grade IIIc lower limb limb injury, according to the Gustilo and Anderson classification, involves an open lower limb fracture with arterial injury requiring repair.

10.39
Answer D
SCC's involving the following sites are listed in order of increasing metastatic potential:
- Sun-exposed sites excluding the lip and ear
- Lip
- Ear
- Non-sun exposed sites
- Marjolin's ulcer

10.40
Answer C
Warthin's tumour is a benign lesion. Ten percent of cases are bilateral. The tumour is commonly found in the tail of the parotid gland.

10.41
Answer B

10.42
Answer D

10.43
Answer B

10.44
Answer G

10.45
Answer E

263

10.46
Answer D

10.47
Answer A

10.48
Answer F

10.49
Answer E

10.50
Answer F

Surgical Educational Applications for the i-Phone and i-Pad produced by

SurgicalIllustration.com

Available from the Apple Apps Store

Surgical Flaps

3D-illustrated animations and diagrams of most commonly used **local flaps** in Plastic Surgery.

Plastic Surgery Quiz

An interactive plastic surgery quiz. The user can set the number of questions and the timing. The quiz maybe done by topics or by choosing to randomize the questions.

Other Titles by
Surgicalillustration.com

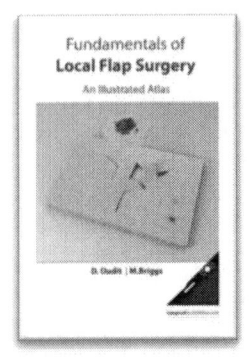

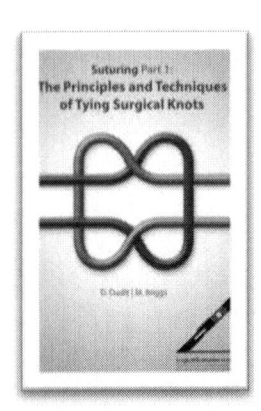

Published by Surgicalillustration.com

Available on Amazon.com

Published by Surgicalillustration.com

Available on Amazon.com

Printed in Great Britain
by Amazon